Intermittent Fasting

Beginners Guide to Weight Loss for Men and Women with Intermittent Fasting

Table of Contents

Introduction 9
Chapter One: History of Intermittent Fasting 10
    Circadian Rhythm and Intermittent Fasting 12
    Gut Microbiome and Intermittent Fasting 13
    Lifestyle Behavior and Intermittent Fasting 13
Chapter Two: Different Methods of Fasting 14
    16/8 Method 14
    The 5:2 Diet 15
    Eat-stop-Eat 15
    Alternate Day Fasting 15
    Warrior Diet 16
    Spontaneous Fasting 16
Chapter Three: Benefits of Intermittent Fasting 17
    Weight loss 17
    Sleep 17
    Resistance to illnesses 17
    A healthy heart 18
    A healthy gut 18
    Tackles diabetes 18
    Reduces inflammation 19
    Promotes cell repair 19
Chapter Four: What to Avoid During a Fast 20
    Who can fast? 20
        Healthy adults 20
        Children 20
        Type-2 diabetes 20
    Who Cannot Fast? 21

Pregnant women 21
Any medical conditions 21
Eating disorders 21
Afraid to fast.. 21
Foods to Avoid and Eat 22
Chapter Five: The Truth about Breakfast............................ 24
Chapter Six: Frequency of Fasting...................................... 27
Skipping breakfast will make you gain weight 27
Your metabolism improves when you eat frequently..... 27
Eating frequently helps keep hunger at bay 28
Small meals assist in weight loss 28
The brain needs glucose constantly 28
Eating often is necessary for good health 29
"Starvation mode" 29
You will lose muscle while fasting................................. 30
It is bad for your health 30
Intermittent Fasting leads to overeating 30
Chapter Seven: Gain Lean Muscle Mass 32
Chapter Eight: How to Get Started 36
Step One: Select a Method 36
Step 2: Research 37
Step 3: Find the necessary tools 37
Step 4: Starting the transition....................................... 37
Step 5: Finding the necessary support.......................... 38
Step 6: Toning down your workouts 38
Step 7: Following delayed gratification......................... 39
Step 8: Protein must be a Priority................................. 39
Step 9: Taking a "before" photograph........................... 40
Step 10: Things to keep in mind.................................... 41

3

- Chapter Nine: Tips and Tricks 42
  - Your mind is the most significant hurdle 44
  - It is easy to lose weight 45
  - If you want, you can build muscle 45
  - You can work while you fast 45
  - Cycle what you eat 46
  - It is a lifestyle 46
  - You will want less food 47
  - Lose fat and gain muscle 47
  - More gains when you fast 48
  - Fasted state 48
  - Drink lots of water 49
  - The best diet 49
- Chapter Ten: Mistakes to Avoid 51
  - Mistake 1: Giving up too soon 51
  - Mistake 2: Binge Eating 51
  - Mistake 3: Not eating enough 51
  - Mistake 4: Wrong Foods 52
  - Mistake 6: Forgetting to drink 52
  - Mistake 7: Taking it too far 53
- Chapter Eleven: Intermittent Fasting and Weight Loss 54
  - Weight Loss 56
  - Resistance or Weight Training 59
  - Cardiovascular Training 60
  - Exercise Intensity and Duration 61
- Chapter Twelve: Intermittent Fasting While Travelling 62
  - Efficiency 62
  - Save money 62
  - Energy 62

    Control 63

    Time 63

    Cleanse 63

Chapter Thirteen: Weight Loss on a Budget 64

    Water, water, and more water 64

    Eat slowly 64

    Eat healthily 65

    Cook at home 65

    Ration your portions 65

    Plan your meals 65

    Grocery shopping 66

    Meal prep 66

    Eat fruit for dessert 66

    Food budget 67

    Eat the healthy stuff first 67

    Brush your teeth after eating 67

    Don't leave the house hungry 68

    Make your snacks 68

    Track what you eat 68

    Exercise 68

Chapter Fourteen: Get Lean while Eating Out 70

    Strategy 1: Nutrition plan 70

    Strategy 2: Stick to the Same Foods 71

    Strategy 3: Increase Protein 71

    Strategy 4: Carbs 71

    Strategy 5: Post Meal Hunger 71

Chapter Fifteen: How to set up a Plan (i.e. 8-Week Meal Plan) 73

    Week One 76

    Week Two' 77

Week Three 77
Week Four 77
Week Five 78
Week Six 78
Week Seven 78
Week Eight 78
Chapter Sixteen: Keeping Up the Motivation 81
Chapter Seventeen: How to Keep the Weight Stable 83
   Skipping breakfast makes you fat 85
   Increase in the frequency of meals helps to boost your metabolism 86
   Eating frequently prevents you from over eating and reduces hunger 86
   Smaller meals can help you lose weight 87
   Your brain requires a constant supply of glucose 87
   Snacking and eating frequently is good for health 88
   Fasting puts your body in starvation mode 89
   Your body is capable of using only a certain amount of protein for each meal 90
   Fasting can make you lose muscle 90
   Fasting is bad for our health 91
   Intermittent Fasting makes us overeat 91
Conclusion 93
Resources 94
Preview of Keto Diet: The Beginners Guide For Men And Women With Ketogenic Diet 95

© **Copyright 2018 by LacoBiz - All rights reserved.**

This document is geared towards providing exact and reliable information in regards to the topic and issue covered. The publication is sold with the idea that the publisher is not required to render accounting, officially permitted, or otherwise, qualified services. If advice is necessary, legal or professional, a practiced individual in the profession should be ordered.

- From a Declaration of Principles which was accepted and approved equally by a Committee of the American Bar Association and a Committee of Publishers and Associations.

In no way is it legal to reproduce, duplicate, or transmit any part of this document in either electronic means or in printed format. Recording of this publication is strictly prohibited and any storage of this document is not allowed unless with written permission from the publisher. All rights reserved.

The information provided herein is stated to be truthful and consistent, in that any liability, in terms of inattention or otherwise, by any usage or abuse of any policies, processes, or directions contained within is the solitary and utter responsibility of the recipient reader. Under no circumstances will any legal responsibility or blame be held against the publisher for any reparation, damages, or monetary loss due to the information herein, either directly or indirectly.

Respective authors own all copyrights not held by the publisher.

The information herein is offered for informational purposes solely, and is universal as so. The presentation of the information is without contract or any type of guarantee assurance.

The trademarks that are used are without any consent, and the publication of the trademark is without permission or backing by the trademark owner. All trademarks and brands within this book are for clarifying purposes only and are the owned by the owners themselves, not affiliated with this document.

Introduction

I want to thank you for choosing the book *"Intermittent Fasting: Beginners Guide to Weight Loss for Men and Women with Intermittent Fasting."*

Do you want a diet that will help you lose weight and improve your overall health? Do you want a diet that doesn't prescribe calorie counting? It does sound quite wonderful if you can achieve your weight loss and health goals without counting calories, doesn't it? If your answer is yes, then you are in for a pleasant surprise! Intermittent Fasting is the diet that you have been looking for. Fasting is not a new concept and has been around for a long time. Intermittent Fasting is a simple variation of fasting and is very helpful. This dieting protocol alternates between periods of fasting and eating.

In this book, you will learn about the basics of Intermittent Fasting, the changes that take place in your body, the benefits it offers, different methods of Intermittent Fasting, tips to exercise, common FAQs and much more. Intermittent Fasting is quite simple. You merely need to make a couple of changes to your eating habits and you are good to go.

If you are fascinated by this diet and want to learn more about it, then let us start right now!

Chapter One: History of Intermittent Fasting

Unlike other forms of conventional dieting, the concept of fasting is quite unambiguous and easy to understand. Did you know that most of us tend to unconsciously follow the protocols of Intermittent Fasting? Do you ever skip having breakfast or dinner? If you do, then you are following an Intermittent Fasting protocol. You will learn about the different methods of Intermittent Fasting in the coming chapters.

Our hunter and gatherer caveman ancestors had to seek food in nature. So, they were often on a fast until they found some nourishment. Then agriculture was introduced, and it led to the formation of human civilization. Whenever there was food scarcity or whenever the seasons changed, fasting was the norm. They used to maintain stocks of grain and meat in cities and castles for harsh winters. Before the introduction of agriculture, shortage of rainfall meant a spell of famine and people used to fast to make their food supplies last longer. Enough rain was quintessential to meet the grain requirement.

Along with civilizations, there came religions. Religions grew when people were living in close quarters and shared similar beliefs. Most of the religions prescribe fasting. Hinduism refers to fasting as Vaasa, and Hindus observe it during festivals or other auspicious days. Fasting is also considered to be a form of penance. Islam prescribes fasting during the holy month of Ramzan. A similar practice is present in Judaism and is known as Yom Kippur. There's a period of fasting before Easter in the Catholic faith.

Technology and innovations play a vital role in the evolution of humans. Industrialization revolutionized the food industry. Mass production of food products meant that the markets were constantly flooded with food products. Apart from this, the way humans view and consume food has also undergone a major change. The human body didn't get a chance to sufficiently adapt itself to the rampant changes brought about by industrialization and agriculture. All this meant that a host of health problems soon followed. Intermittent Fasting is quite an old practice. Even though it is an old practice, humans have just begun to understand and truly appreciate the various benefits this diet offers. Whenever you fast, you give your body a chance to cleanse itself - not just cleanse but even repair and regenerate itself from within.

Essentially, while fasting your body gets to burn out all the excess fat it has stored. Human beings have evolved in such a manner that we can fast without any health risks and that is normal. Body fat is the reserve of food that the body has stashed away for a rainy day. If you don't consume food, your body will simply reach into this reserve to provide you with energy. There needs to be balance in everything you do. There's a yin and a yang. The same rule applies to eating and fasting as well. Fasting is the flip side of eating. If you aren't eating, then you are fasting. When you eat something, this leads to an accumulation of food energy that isn't going to be made use of immediately. A portion of this is stored away. A hormone known as insulin is responsible for storing the food energy. When you eat something, there is a spike in the level of insulin. This facilitates the storage of energy in two different ways. Sugars are linked into long chains and this is known as glycogen. The rest is stored in the liver. When the space available has been maxed out, the liver starts turning the rest into fat. Some of this fat so created is stored in the liver and the rest is stored in the form of fat cells in the rest of your body. There isn't a limit on fat creation. So, there are two forms of energy stores in our bodies. One is easily accessible and has a limited storage space (glycogen), and the other is the harder to reach energy without a limit on storage (body fat).

This process is essentially reversed when you don't eat, that is during fasting. There will be a reduction in the level of insulin and this enables your body to reach into its storage of fat cells and burn this to provide energy. The most easily attainable source of energy for your body is glycogen. This is broken down into molecules of glucose that sustains your body. This can provide sufficient energy for your body to function for 24 hours or longer. After this, your body will reach into its fat reserves to generate energy. Your body will do this only while feeding or fasting. Either your body will be storing energy, or it will be burning energy. Only either of these processes can take place at any given time. If there is a balance between eating and fasting, then there will not be any weight gain. Over a period of time, you will start gaining weight if you haven't given your body sufficient time to burn all the food it has stored. To restore balance, you will need to give your body sufficient time to burn the food energy. This can be accomplished by fasting. This is how our bodies are designed. Intermittent Fasting helps to restore this much-needed balance.

Circadian Rhythm and Intermittent Fasting

Human beings, like other organisms, have a biological circadian clock that ensures that the physiological processes in the body are performed at the right time. The circadian rhythm is on all day long and it affects the biology and the behavior of humans. Any disruption in this rhythm has a negative effect on the metabolism and it can cause several metabolic dysfunctions like obesity, diabetes and a host of cardiovascular diseases. The primary factor that affects the circadian rhythm is the signal to eat. It is responsible for metabolic, physiological and behavioral pathways in the body. All these pathways are responsible for making sure that your body performs optimally. Apart from this, they also ensure that your body is healthy. You can use behavioral intervention to regulate the body's circadian rhythm. Yes, you guessed it right! Intermittent Fasting is a means of behavioral intervention that will streamline the circadian rhythm. This in turn leads to better gene expression and improvement in your body's health and metabolism.

Gut Microbiome and Intermittent Fasting

The gastrointestinal tract regulates multiple processes within your body. In other words, your gut helps regulate different physiological and biochemical functions in your body. For instance, the metabolic reaction to glucose and the blood flow are higher during the day than at night. Even a small fluctuation in the circadian rhythm can impair your metabolism and increases the risk of several chronic diseases. The microbiome present in the gut is usually referred to as the second brain. It is known as the second brain because of the influence it has over your metabolism and physiology. Intermittent Fasting has a positive impact on the gut microbiome. It makes the gut less permeable, reduces the chances of systemic inflammation and improves overall energy balance.

Lifestyle Behavior and Intermittent Fasting

Intermittent Fasting helps change different health-related behaviors like calorie consumption, energy expenditure and your sleep cycle. Therefore, it is not a surprise that these are the three primary functions that help fight the most significant health concern that plagues the human community, obesity. You will learn more about the different benefits it offers in the coming chapters.

Chapter Two: Different Methods of Fasting

Intermittent Fasting is a varied and a dynamic diet that offers multiple health benefits. There are different methods of Intermittent Fasting that you can follow, and you need to select one that will meet your needs. So, read on to learn more about the different methods of Intermittent Fasting.

16/8 Method

If you follow this method of Intermittent Fasting, you must fast for 16 hours daily. If you fast for 16 hours, the eating window comes down to 8 hours. You can squeeze in two or three healthy meals within this time frame. It is popularly known as the LeanGains method. The creator of this variant of Intermittent Fasting was Martin Berkhan, a fitness expert. This method can be something as simple as skipping your breakfast and directly having your first meal at noon and your last one at about 8 p.m.

The next meal you can have will be on the following day at noon. So, you will fast for 16 hours and, frankly, you will not even feel like you were fasting for 16 hours. Ideally, women must not fast for more than 14 hours. If you like to wake up early and eat breakfast, then have a hearty breakfast, then you need to make sure that your last meal is at around 4 or 6 in the evening.

You are free to consume all sorts of calorie-free beverages throughout the day like water, black coffee or any other herbal teas. You need to make sure that you don't include any sugar in your drinks, since it will effectively break your fast. If you want to lose weight, then you must not binge on junk foods when you break your fast. This method works, only if you strictly follow the protocols of the diet.

The 5:2 Diet

In this variation of the diet, you need to restrict your calorie intake on two days of the week and eat like you normally do on the other days. On the days you need to restrict your calorie intake, the calories you consume must be between 500 and 600. Michael Mosley is the creator of this diet and it is also known as the Fast diet. On the days that you fast, you must ensure you don't consume more than 600 calories. You can squeeze in two small meals within this calorie limit. This diet is ideal for all those who don't like the idea of fasting daily.

Eat-stop-Eat

In this form of Intermittent Fasting, you must fast for 24 hours, once or twice in a week. Brad Pilon, a famous fitness expert, created this diet.

You can choose the days you want to fast on. For instance, if your fast starts at 8 p.m. on Monday night, then you will break your fast only at 8 p.m. on Tuesday night. You can decide when you want to fast, if you fast for 24-hours. You cannot consume any solid food during your fasting period but can have calorie-free beverages. You must ensure that you are consuming healthy meals on the normal days. If you are just getting started with fasting, then this might be a little complicated. Instead, it is a good idea to start with either of the previous methods and then make your way toward this dieting protocol. If you want to follow this diet, then you need self-discipline and self-control.

Make sure that your fasting period never exceeds 48 hours. So, don't try to fast on two days continuously and pace it evenly.

Alternate Day Fasting

If you want to follow this method of Intermittent Fasting, then you need to consume 500 calories on every alternate day. If you are not a fan of a strict diet, then this will work well for you. You can eat like you normally do on all days except for the ones with the calorie restriction.

Warrior Diet

Ori Hofmekler, a famous fitness expert, was the creator of this diet. In this method, you need to have small portions of raw fruits and vegetables during the day and end your day with a hearty meal at night. You will essentially be fasting throughout the day and will feast at night. The eating window in this method is restricted to about 4 hours. The food that you can consume on this diet is quite like the food you can consume while following a Paleo diet. So, you are free to fill up on foods that are unprocessed. It essentially means that you can eat only those foods that our cavemen ancestors had access to. If you feel like your caveman ancestors could not have eaten something, then neither can you. If you don't want to fast all day long, you can snack on fruit and vegetables. It will keep your hunger pangs at bay.

Spontaneous Fasting

As the name suggests, you merely need to skip meals spontaneously. There is no fixed plan. If you don't feel like eating, you simply need to skip a meal. There will be times when you don't have time to eat or when you don't feel like eating. So, whenever you skip a meal, you are effectively following the protocols of this diet. It will not do your body any harm if you skip meals from time to time.

Chapter Three: Benefits of Intermittent Fasting

Perhaps the most common reason why people opt for Intermittent Fasting is to lose weight. Apart from weight loss, there are various other benefits this diet offers, and you will learn about them in this chapter.

Weight loss

Intermittent Fasting alternates between periods of eating and fasting. If you fast, naturally your calorie intake will reduce, and it also helps you maintain your weight loss. It also prevents you from indulging in mindless eating. Whenever you eat something, your body converts the food into glucose and fat. It uses the glucose immediately and stores the fat for later use. When you skip a few meals, your body starts to reach into its internal stores of fat to provide energy. As soon as your body starts burning fats due to the shortage of glucose, you will start to lose weight. Also, most of the fat that you lose is from the abdominal region. If you want a flat tummy, then this is the perfect diet for you.

Sleep

Lack of sleep is a primary cause of obesity. When your body doesn't get enough sleep, the internal mechanism of burning fat suffers. Intermittent Fasting regulates your sleep cycle and, in turn, it makes your body effectively burn fats. A good sleep cycle has different physiological benefits - it makes you feel energetic and elevates your overall mood.

Resistance to illnesses

Intermittent Fasting helps in the growth and the regeneration of cells. Did you know that the human body has an internal mechanism that helps repair damaged cells? Intermittent

Fasting helps kickstart this mechanism. It improves the overall functioning of all the cells in the body. So, it is directly responsible for improving your body's natural defense mechanism by increasing its resistance to diseases and illnesses.

A healthy heart

Intermittent Fasting assists in weight loss, and weight loss improves your cardiovascular health. A buildup of plaque in blood vessels is known as atherosclerosis. This is the primary cause for various cardiovascular diseases. Endothelium is the thin lining of blood vessels and any dysfunction in it results in atherosclerosis. Obesity is the primary problem that plagues humanity and is also the main reason for the increase of plaque deposits in the blood vessels. Stress and inflammation also increase the severity of this problem. Intermittent Fasting tackles the buildup of fat and helps tackle obesity. So, all you need to do is follow the simple protocols of Intermittent Fasting to improve your overall health.

A healthy gut

There are several millions of microorganisms present in your digestive system. These microorganisms help improve the overall functioning of your digestive system and are known as gut microbiome. Intermittent Fasting improves the health of these microbiome and improves your digestive health. A healthy digestive system helps in better absorption of food and improves the functioning of your stomach.

Tackles diabetes

Diabetes is a serious problem on its own. It is also a primary indicator of the increase in risk factors of various cardiovascular diseases like heart attacks and strokes. When the glucose level increases alarmingly in the bloodstream and there isn't enough insulin to process this glucose, it causes diabetes. When the body is resistant to insulin, it becomes difficult to regulate the insulin levels in the body. Intermittent Fasting reduces insulin sensitivity and helps tackle diabetes.

Reduces inflammation

Whenever your body feels there is an internal problem, its natural defense is inflammation. It doesn't mean that all forms of inflammation are desirable. Inflammation can cause several serious health conditions like arthritis, atherosclerosis and other neurodegenerative disorders.

Any inflammation of this nature is known as chronic inflammation and is quite painful. Chronic inflammation can restrict your body's movements too. If you want to keep inflammation in check, then Intermittent Fasting will certainly come in handy.

Promotes cell repair

When you fast, the cells in your body start the process of waste removal. Waste removal means the breaking down of all dysfunctional cells and proteins and is known as autophagy. Autophagy offers protection against several degenerative diseases like Alzheimer's and cancer. You don't like accumulating garbage in your home, do you? Similarly, your body must not hold onto any unnecessary toxins. Autophagy is the body's way of getting rid of all things unnecessary.

Chapter Four: What to Avoid During a Fast

Intermittent Fasting helps rectify and reverse several health conditions, but it doesn't mean that it is ideal for everyone. An important thing that you need to keep in mind is that you need to consult your medical practitioner before you start this diet.

Who can fast?

The following people can fast

Healthy adults

All healthy adults can fast. It helps cleanse the body and there aren't any reasons why a healthy adult cannot fast.

Children

Usually, it isn't suitable for children up to the age of 18 to fast; however, children can fast. A child must only fast for a short duration and must not fast for prolonged periods. A perfectly healthy child doesn't have to fast. The general exception to this rule is all those who suffer from obesity. A child needs plenty of nutrition for growth and their body needs nourishment constantly. If the child is less than 18 years, please consult a medical practitioner.

Type-2 diabetes

Fasting helps reverse the harmful effects of type-2 diabetes. If you suffer from this, then you are free to fast. Before you start any diet, you must always consult your medical practitioner.

Who Cannot Fast?

Pregnant women

As such, there is no conclusive proof that shows the effect of Intermittent Fasting on a fetus. It is better to abstain from any diets if you are pregnant or are trying to conceive. If you are planning to start a family, then your body needs plenty of nutrition and you must not restrict your diet at this point of time. Also, mothers who are breast-feeding need to abstain from Intermittent Fasting. Fasting reduces the nutrition available in breast milk and it also affects the quantity of milk that is produced.

Any medical conditions

If you have any health concerns related to the kidney or the liver, then you must not fast. You need to consult a doctor before you fast if you have any pre-existing medical conditions. If you use any medication for high blood pressure or have a weak immune system, then you must not fast. You can fast even if you have medical conditions, but don't forget to consult your doctor.

If you have recently had a major surgery, then please abstain from fasting. Also, fasting is not ideal for all those who are recovering from any major illness.

Eating disorders

If you have any eating disorders or are recovering from an eating disorder, then you must not fast. Fasting can cause a relapse and you need to avoid it at any cost.

Afraid to fast

If fasting scares you, then don't fast. Fear is an unnecessary stressor and it will just cause problems. Fear is a powerful emotion and can alter your psychological makeup. If you think you cannot handle fasting, then don't try to fast. If you want this diet to generate positive results, you need to have an open mindset!

Foods to Avoid and Eat

When you are following the protocols of Intermittent Fasting, the primary focus is not on what you eat, but it is on when you eat. Just because it doesn't focus on what you eat, it doesn't mean that you stuff yourself with carbs and sugar-laden treats. For best results, it is a good idea to stay away from all processed foods and opt for healthy foods. It means that it is a good idea to avoid all sugary treats or at least try to limit them as much as you possibly can. So, avoid cookies, chocolates, cakes, and all packaged sweets.

Stay away from foods rich in unhealthy fats and carbs like burgers, pizzas and all fast foods. Say no to foods that are devoid of all protein and are full of sugars and carbs. Avoid soy products if you want to lose weight. Soy products are rich in estrogen and a high level of estrogen will not do you any good.

You need to maintain a calorie deficit if you want to lose weight. The higher the level of insulin in your body, the less fat you will lose. Carbs and sugars increase the level of insulin. So, if you want to regulate your insulin levels, you need to avoid carbs.

There are some people who believe that you can eat a lot of protein, fruit and vegetables while fasting. If you eat all this during a fast, you aren't effectively fasting, are you? Even if you had a couple of drops of honey to your morning tea, you will be effectively breaking your fast. Just because you aren't permitted to eat anything, doesn't mean that you stop drinking water.

Your body needs at least 8 glasses of water to stay hydrated and ensure that you are thoroughly hydrated. Drinking water will make you feel fuller and helps you to avoid any hunger pangs.

You are free to consume all calorie-free beverages like black tea, black coffee, green tea, herbal teas and carbonated water. Try to limit your caffeine intake. Caffeine has a diuretic effect on the body and too much of it can cause dehydration due to the loss of electrolytes. Try to limit your caffeine intake to about two cups of coffee or any other caffeinated calorie-free drink of your choice. It might seem quite tempting to add some sugar or cream to your coffee, or perhaps some honey to your tea. If you do this, you will cause a spike in your insulin levels. When there is a spike in your insulin levels, your body stops burning fat and it negates the benefits of fasting. You must try to avoid anything that will cause a spike in your insulin levels and effectively break your fast. Some people believe that chewing sugar-free gum will keep hunger at bay. Even all those products that are labeled as "no sugar" or "sugar-free" include some carbs in them.

If you really want to lose weight and want to improve your overall health, then it is a good idea to stay away from all forms of alcoholic drinks as well. Alcohol contains a lot of carbs that can sneak up on you unknowingly. Intermittent Fasting helps cleanse your body. So, if you really want to cleanse your body then you need to avoid all the things that will result in the internal buildup of toxins. So, stay away from alcohol to improve the efficiency of this diet.

Chapter Five: The Truth about Breakfast

Losing weight can be a little tricky at times. Do you want to know if you can speed up this process and effectively turn your body into a fat burning machine? If yes, then you need to start skipping breakfast. Yes, you read it right. You might think this isn't a good idea since breakfast is the most important meal of the day. Well, hold your horses before you jump to any conclusions. Go through the information given in this chapter and it will certainly change your beliefs about breakfast.

The human physiology is based on the feast-famine pattern of eating; the basic hunter-gatherer nature of our homo-sapien ancestors is still present within us. We might live in a modern world where there is dearth of food, but our bodies didn't have the necessary time to get used to this change. The constant dilemma that exists between modern society and our basic physiology is not a new problem. It isn't a good idea to ignore our basic physiology. Instead, you need to try to understand it so that you can do all that is necessary to make the most of your metabolism. If you want your body to work for you, then you need to take the time to understand how it works. You need to work with your metabolism and not against it, if you want to achieve your weight loss and health goals.

It is a popular belief that breakfast is the most important meal of the day. Almost all the popular weight-loss protocols recommend consuming a hearty breakfast. Another popular myth that we all seem to believe to be true is that skipping breakfast will cause obesity. Well, where did all these so-called truths come from? If you take a moment and think about it, these statements will not make any sense to you.

How can you even put on weight if you restrict your calorie intake? What is essential for weight loss? The answer is calorie deficit. So, if you skip breakfast, your body is in a calorie deficit and that must promote weight loss. So, doesn't it seem absurd to believe that skipping breakfast will make you gain weight?

So, it is nothing more than a myth and skipping breakfast will not make you fat. In fact, as per research published in 2014 in the *American Journal of Clinical Nutrition, this* showed that eating or skipping breakfast has no effect on weight loss.

When it comes to consuming food, the one thing you must never forget is to listen to your body. Your body is quite smart, and it knows what it wants. So, you must eat only when you are hungry. When your body needs food, it will let you know. If you don't feel hungry in the morning, then don't force yourself to eat breakfast and simply skip that meal. It is perfectly normal to skip breakfast and a lot of people do this.

Did you ever wonder why you don't feel hungry in the morning? The circadian system keeps our bodies in sync with the 24-hour format of day and night and our response to light and darkness. The Circadian system also affects your hormones, digestion and body temperature. Apart from this, it controls your hunger or appetite and is responsible for the lack of hunger in the morning and the hunger pangs in the evening. If you fast all night long, then you will not be hungry in the morning.

If there is a constant supply of glucose, then your body will not burn fat. Glucose is the easiest form of energy for your body and it will not tap into your fat reserves if you constantly give it glucose as a choice. If you keep consuming five or six meals a day, you will not burn any fats. You need to restrict your food intake if you want your body to burn fats.

All the food that you consume is converted into glucose and excess glucose is stored within the cells in the form of fat molecules. When you restrict your food intake for prolonged periods like you do while on Intermittent Fasting, then your body starts to reach into its fat stores to provide energy. You can optimize this process of burning fats by postponing your first meal of the day.

It is a common misconception that your body needs constant supply of glucose to function optimally. It might be true if you suffer from low sugar levels, but if you are healthy adult, then you don't have to worry about this. You don't have to keep eating after every couple of hours. If you keep feeding your body all the time, it starts to become resistant to insulin and it causes a whole range of health problems.

In fact, the most popular method of Intermittent Fasting-LeanGains, recommends that you skip breakfast. When you are asleep, your body keeps producing certain hormones that process fat and store some energy. So, as soon as you wake up in the morning, you will feel a burst of energy! This energy can keep you going for a couple of hours at least! You don't have to worry about skipping breakfast and it will certainly not harm you.

Chapter Six: Frequency of Fasting

Intermittent Fasting is a pattern of eating that oscillates between periods of eating and fasting. There are a lot of myths about this method of fasting. In this chapter, let us debunk the most popular misconceptions that exist about fasting, snacking, and the frequency of eating.

Skipping breakfast will make you gain weight

Well, breakfast isn't as important as people seem to think. It might be thought of as the most important meal of the day, but it really isn't, and that notion is just a myth. People believe that skipping breakfast leads to excessive hunger and weight gain. There are no scientific studies or research that supports this claim. Skipping breakfast won't make you fat and you can do so quite safely without any fear. You can fast for 16 to 24 hours at a stretch without worrying about the functioning of your body. Your body knows what's best for it so trust your body.

Your metabolism improves when you eat frequently

It is a popular myth that eating frequently helps improve your metabolism. Eating small meals does not improve your body's ability to burn calories. Yes, your body does need some energy to digest and assimilate the food you consume. This is referred to as thermic effect of food and it accounts for about 20-30% of total calories from protein, 5-10% from carbs and about 3% from fats. On an average, the thermic effect of food accounts for 10% of the total calories you consume. You need to take into consideration the total calories you consume and not the number of meals you eat. You don't need to keep eating constantly. For instance, if you have three meals of 1000 calories each the thermic effect will be 300 calories and it will be the same if you have 6 meals of 500 calories each. So, you can fast for prolonged periods of time and not worry about slowing down your body's metabolism.

Eating frequently helps keep hunger at bay

People believe that snacking constantly helps to keep hunger at bay and reduces the chances of excessive hunger. Frequent meals will obviously leave you feeling full, but you don't have to do this. If you want to reduce your cravings and keep hunger at bay, then you need to make sure that you are filling yourself up with the right kind of food. Your meals must contain high amounts of fiber, protein and healthy fats instead of carbs. A meal that's rich in carbs will make you feel hungry soon and make you want to eat more food. Consuming carbs makes you crave for carbs. So, a balanced meal is the key to reducing your hunger. You don't have to worry about hungry pangs while following the protocols of Intermittent Fasting.

Small meals assist in weight loss

As mentioned earlier, frequent meals don't help boost your metabolism. Small meals won't do your body any good and they certainly don't help in weight loss. Eating frequently has the opposite of the desired effect. You can fast for an entire day without worrying about your body metabolism. There won't be a change in your energy levels if you keep snacking constantly. If you are worried that fasting leads to weight gain, you can lay those fears to rest. In fact, your body will start burning its reserves of fat to provide energy if you restrict the supply of glucose.

The brain needs glucose constantly

Yes, the brain does need glucose to function. This doesn't mean that you need to keep consuming carbs every couple of hours for our brain to keep functioning. It certainly won't stop functioning if you don't eat anything for an extended period. This misconception is due to the assumption that the brain needs glucose to function. Even if you restrict the consumption of food, your body can burn fats and produce energy that will keep your body going. Your body starts producing glucose that's necessary by a process known as gluconeogenesis. There is a reserve of glucose in the body and your liver breaks this down to supply glucose that is essential for the functioning of your brain. Even during the 24-hour format of fasting, your brain will function, and you don't have to worry about that. The dietary fats present in the body will be broken down into ketones by the liver for supplying the necessary energy your body needs. Ketones help in the functioning of the brain. Think about this from an evolutionary point of view. Human beings might have become extinct a long time ago if carbs were the only way for our survival. However, if an individual has hypoglycemia, then they will need to snack after every couple of hours if they don't want to get sick.

Eating often is necessary for good health

Being in a constantly fed state isn't natural for the human body. During evolution, humans had to endure periods of starvation. If eating often was essential for survival, then human beings might have been wiped out a long time ago. In fact, fasting helps to induce cellular repair by kick starting the process of autophagy. This helps to provide protection against diseases like Alzheimer's and even certain types of cancer. Fasting is quite beneficial for the system and it helps cleanse the system by eliminating the build-up of toxins in the body. Snacking often has certain disadvantages as well. Frequent meals increase your calorie intake and lead to a build-up of fatty cells in the liver. This doesn't do your body any good.

"Starvation mode"

A popular argument against Intermittent Fasting is that it puts your body into starvation mode. While fasting, the body assumes that it's starving, and therefore shuts down its metabolism and prevents the burning of fat to produce energy. Long-term weight loss reduces the calories you burn and that's what starvation mode is. However, this is bound to happen regardless of the dieting protocol you follow. Short-term fasting helps speed up the metabolic function of the body. The increase in the levels of noradrenaline in the body increases the break down of the fat cells and thereby boosts the metabolism as well. Fasting for up to 48 hours helps boost the metabolism, but anything more than this reverses this effect. You can fast if you follow a sensible fasting protocol.

You will lose muscle while fasting

Once again, it is nothing more than a misconception that fasting leads to muscle loss. Fasting leads to fat loss and nothing else. In fact, Intermittent Fasting helps to increase the build-up of lean muscle and when coupled with the right exercises, it helps build muscle. Continuous calorie restriction for days on end leads to the loss of muscle. However, this isn't the case with Intermittent Fasting and you don't have to worry about losing muscle. You will learn more about building muscle in the coming chapters.

It is bad for your health

Some believe that fasting is harmful. Intermittent Fasting has several health benefits and these claims can be backed by scientific research. So, thinking that fasting is bad for overall wellbeing is nothing but a myth and it must not be taken seriously. In the previous chapter, the different health benefits of Intermittent Fasting were explained in detail. So, do you still think this diet is bad for you after going through the list of benefits it offers? Clearly this is just a myth and you must not pay any heed to it.

Intermittent Fasting leads to overeating

Some claim that Intermittent Fasting doesn't lead to weight loss and that instead it leads to overeating. After a fast, your consumption of food might be slightly higher. But this wears off quite quickly. Once your body gets acclimatized to prolonged periods of fasting, your calorie intake will start decreasing. You won't try to compensate for your fasting period by eating more during your eating window. Your body will slowly get used to fasting and you certainly don't have to worry about putting on weight.

Fasting certainly isn't bad for you and it can help improve your overall health. Depending on the Intermittent Fasting protocol that you opt for, your fasting schedule will change. You don't have to worry about the frequency of fasting, since your body will get the nutrients it needs to function properly.

Chapter Seven: Gain Lean Muscle Mass

There has been an ongoing debate about whether it is good to exercise on an empty stomach or not. This heated debate has been going on since weights were introduced in gyms. As mentioned, it is a heated discussion and different people have different opinions. In this section, you will learn about how you can improve the efficiency of your workouts while on this diet.

One of the first things that we need to do is get some clarity about small and frequent meals. The popular opinion about eating smaller and frequent meals seems to be that it helps to speed up the metabolism and assists in burning fat. People also seem to think that it promotes the growth of muscle. You need to understand that there isn't the necessary research that supports these claims. Another idea that needs some clarification is whether it is a good idea to work out on empty stomach or not. The last question that needs some clarification is whether skipping meals will slow down your metabolism and increase the desire to eat.

You might wonder how you can clarify all these opposing opinions. Well, there are certain beliefs about Intermittent Fasting. You will learn about all these opinions and the facts related to these opinions that will help you. In this chapter, you will learn about exercising while following the protocols of Intermittent Fasting.

An empty stomach results in certain hormonal changes within your body that can promote the burning of stored fats and the building of muscle. An empty stomach increases your body's sensitivity to insulin and increases the production of growth hormones.

The Pancreas produces insulin in your body and it helps your body process the food that you consume. Insulin removes the blood sugar from your bloodstream and it transports it to the fat cells, muscles and liver for use later. The problem starts when you eat too much and too frequently, all this decreases the sensitivity of your body to insulin. A lower level of insulin sensitivity brings a host of health troubles like the inability to lose weight, gain weight, increase the fat content and increases the risk of several cardiovascular diseases along the way. If you eat less frequently, like you will while on Intermittent Fasting, it reduces the production of insulin and, therefore, lowers the risk of insulin sensitivity. The less insulin your body produces, the more sensitive it becomes to insulin and it helps burn the stored fat and reduces the risk of diabetes and cardiovascular disease.

When you exercise on empty stomach, your body pumps up the production of the magic elixir known as growth hormone that's necessary for the growth of muscles, stronger bones, longevity and for better fat burning. Some studies show that a 24-hour fast can increase the production of growth hormone in men by up to 2000% and by up to 1300% in women. These numbers seem quite unbelievable, don't they? All this by merely fasting for 24-hours.

You might be curious about the intermittent protocol and if it will affect your muscle mass. You will still be able to build muscle while following this diet. There are three things that you will need to keep in mind. Read on to learn more.

The Intermittent Fasting method that you might opt for will depend on the kind of a lifestyle that you are leading. Depending on your needs, whether spiritual or physical, you can select a specific method of fasting. Regardless of your reasons for starting on this diet, you might be wondering how you can build muscle while following the Intermittent Fasting protocols. It is a general misconception that you won't be able to build any muscle, but this cannot be further away from truth. There are a couple of things that you can do to maximize your success.

If you have a specific time when you are fasting, let's assume from 5 in the morning until 7 at night, then it is ideal if you can squeeze working out into your schedule during the evening hours. Waking up earlier than 5 a.m. isn't really possible. You will also need to eat before engaging in resistance training. So, working out in the middle of the day isn't advisable. You will need to consume proteins and carbs after working out to kickstart the recovery process. If you are training in the evening, then you can squeeze in a small meal after working out. You can work out for an hour and still give your body some time to recover before going to sleep.

You must plan your meals in such a way that the bulk of the calories you are supposed to consume is eaten right after your workout. It is important that you do this, because at this point your body will utilize all these calories to produce lean muscle mass and it will also facilitate in the recovery process. You will need to figure out the number of calories that you will need for building muscle. You will need to consume 20% of those calories prior to working out. The calories you consume must be a mix of proteins and carbohydrates. The other 60% of the total calories must be consumed in the period following your workout. You can spread this over two small meals if you want to and distribute it over the next couple of hours. Your calorie intake will definitely be high, and you can get in as many calories as you can by opting for foods that are rich in calories like oats, red meats and so on. Make sure that you are consuming foods that are rich in carbs after your workout. It will provide your body with the necessary calories to kick start the recovery process. You needn't worry about eliminating all fats from your meals. Instead, you can consume a large meal that's rich in carbs or proteins immediately after your training session and then have a high fat or protein meal just before you go to sleep. You must make it a point that your post-workout meal has low fat content. Fats are rich in calories and it is easier to have them in higher volumes (nuts, oils, and so on). It is certainly easier to have these than shoveling down carbs when you are already feeling full.

Finally, there is one more thing that you must keep in mind while following Intermittent Fasting protocols if you want to build some muscle. As soon as you wake up, you must eat something. If you are just fasting for the sake of convenience, then you must eat something according to your usual time of waking up in the morning. You must consume something just before your fast starts. Have some protein that can be digested slowly like red meat and cottage cheese. This meal must account for 20% of your daily calorie intake. A few carbs and fat can also be added to this meal. It will provide your body with the necessary amino acids to get through your fasting period. You have the option of going back to sleep if you feel like it. Having to wake up to eat and then going back to sleep is a hassle. This isn't something that will be sustainable in the long run. You must plan in such a manner that your body will get used to this schedule of eating. If you are used to waking up early in the morning, then this will be quite simple. You won't have to make any extra adjustments to your schedule. It will fit right in.

Make sure that you keep these tips in mind. If you try to engage in high intensity workouts while maintaining a low-calorie intake due to prolonged periods of fasting, this idea is likely to backfire. You will end up tiring yourself and your body will not have the necessary glucose to start the recovery process. After a while, your body will be depleted of glycogen and this will not do you any good. To prevent this, you will need to get used to eating forcefully. Your body will get used to this after a while, and it will start feeling normal. So, be patient and give yourself some time to get used to it.

Chapter Eight: How to Get Started

Well, now that you know what Intermittent Fasting is all about and how it works, the next step is for you to get started with this diet. Intermittent Fasting is not merely a dieting protocol, but it is a way of life. Intermittent Fasting is sustainable in the long run and isn't a short-term diet. If you want to achieve and maintain your weight loss and overall health, then you must stick to this diet. Intermittent Fasting will help you shed all those extra kilos you want to lose. In this section, you will learn about the different steps that you can follow to get started on this diet.

Staring a new diet might seem slightly intimidating, but with the help of these steps, it will not seem intimidating.

Step One: Select a Method

There are various types of Intermittent Fasting protocols that you can choose from. One of the most versatile patterns of dieting these days is Intermittent Fasting. You need to opt for a method that fits your lifestyle, personality and meets your goals. If you are used to waking up early and like exercising, then the method of Intermittent Fasting that you can opt for is the 16:8 method. If you select this method, then you can have a breakfast in the morning and have your last meal in the evening. If you are used to skipping breakfast or don't mind skipping breakfast, then you can have your first meal at noon and your last meal at night. If you don't like the idea of fasting daily, then you can choose the alternate day fasting protocol and fast on alternate days. The method that you opt for is entirely up to you. You can customize this diet to meet your requirements. There is a method of fasting that will meet your requirements and you merely need to make up your mind about the method you want to opt for.

Step 2: Research

Go through all the information that is given in this book before you decide to select a specific method. Always select a method that suits your lifestyle. If you do this, it will be quite easy to stick to your dieting protocol. When compared to other conventional diets, this method is quite relaxed since Intermittent Fasting doesn't place much emphasis on what you eat but instead concentrates on when you eat. Check your priorities and find a method that will suit your needs. Once you establish your goals, you need to research about the fasting protocol you want to opt for. If you want to lose fat and gain lean muscle, then the method you must opt for is LeanGains.

Step 3: Find the necessary tools

There are various apps that you can use to help you with this diet. You can choose from free as well as paid applications to track your progress. Intermittent Fasting is essentially a method of trial and error. One method might be quite effective for some while something else might work for others. You can download an application that will help track your progress and determine whether a specific method is effective or not. If you want to, you can also maintain a food journal to track your progress. You need to make a note of when you eat and what you eat, along with the progress you are making.

Step 4: Starting the transition

Starting this diet might be a little tricky, if you don't have an all or nothing attitude. If you are used to skipping meals every now and then, then Intermittent Fasting will be quite simple. If you are not used to fasting and have never fasted before, then it will be a little difficult until you gain some footing. You need to prepare yourself mentally for the diet you want to follow. It might seem a little daunting that you need to go for prolonged periods without eating. Well, the one thing that you need to remember is that all your fears are baseless and, in fact, there is nothing that you need to fear. The fear is in your head and you will not get over it unless you take the first step.

You need to take some time to condition your body. To condition your body, you can slowly start increasing the gap between two meals. After you do this, you can start by slowly skipping a meal a day so that your body gets used to the idea of fasting. If you are used to snacking between meals, then you can slowly cut down on snacks. Instead, you can start filling yourself up with foods that will leave you feeling fuller for longer. After you do this, you can start with a relatively easy method of fasting. You can start with the alternate-day fasting method or the LeanGains method. It is all about slowly conditioning yourself to the diet and the idea of dieting. Once you do this, you will be able to follow the diet rather easily.

Step 5: Finding the necessary support

Everyone needs a support system. Your support system will encourage you and motivate you to keep going even when you feel like giving up. You can also start your diet with a diet buddy or partner. Find a partner for yourself and start the diet together. Your dieting buddy can be your partner, spouse, friend or anyone else. You can each use the other as a coach and a mentor along the way. If you cannot find someone to do this with, then you can explain your situation to someone and make them hold you accountable for the progress you make. Make that person check on you and the progress you are making.

Step 6: Toning down your workouts

You need to tone down your workout routine, at least initially. You need to give your body some time to get used to the new diet before you can go back to your exercise routine. When your body is getting used to a new diet, it is quite likely that you might feel a little low on energy. In such a situation, if you push yourself too hard, you risk burning yourself out and it will not do you any good.

Step 7: Following delayed gratification

Delayed gratification is a brilliant technique and it works rather well with this form of dieting. There might be times when a hunger pang strikes you and you might start craving for something sweet. Whenever this happens, make a list of the things that you want to eat. Keep adding the items to this list whenever you feel hungry. When this happens, you need to tell yourself that you cannot eat that right now and you can eat it later. When you do this, it helps to stop your mind about obsessing over things that you must not eat. You need to control your mind and you must not let it control you. You need to eat only those foods that are good for you.

Step 8: Protein must be a Priority

Always make sure that you eat the necessary proteins and complex carbs before anything else. You might have something sweet or oily on your eating list, but all that can wait. If you give in to your urge to eat something you aren't supposed to, then you will end up overeating. Also, it is quite likely that you will fill yourself up with junk during the eating window and then experience hunger pangs when you start fasting. When you are eating, you need to understand that you are prepping your body for the fasting period. So, you must always eat those foods that will leave you feeling fuller for longer like proteins, healthy carbs and dietary fats.

If you start feeling hungry while fasting, it is likely that you will give up on your diet. To avoid this, eat healthy and wholesome meals.

Avoid all sorts of processed foods that are full of sugars, unhealthy fats, and undesirable carbs. Instead, opt for healthy foods that are rich in fiber, nutrients, and the essential macros.

Healthy food will nourish your body and will leave you feeling energetic. Unhealthy foods like chocolates or chips can be replaced with some fruits or nuts. Here are a couple of simple tips that you can keep in mind to make sure that you are eating wholesome food.

Have complex carbohydrates like whole grains and leafy vegetables instead of starchy foods like bread, pasta or pizza. Your meal must be rich in protein because it not only leaves you feeling fuller for longer, but it is good for you as well. Stay away from all processed foods and opt for healthy treats like kale chips, nuts, fruits, or anything that isn't full of saturated fats and trans fats. Replace sugary drinks with water (sparkling or still). Create a food plan for yourself. If you are interested in cooking, then learn to experiment with recipes and cook something different. Healthy food doesn't mean bland salads, so keep an open mind and try your hand at cooking. If you plan your meals in advance, then you can do all the meal prep on your day off, this does simplify the entire cooking process.

Step 9: Taking a "before" photograph

Before you start following any of the protocols of Intermittent Fasting, there is one little step along the way that you need to take. You need to take a photograph of yourself. You can label it as a "before" photograph. This will help you to get started. If you follow the protocols of Intermittent Fasting properly, then you will be able to see a positive change in your body. Keep taking a weekly photograph of yourself and make a timeline of the photographs. It will help you see the progress you are making. At times, you might need a little extra motivation to keep going. Whenever you hit a snag, you simply need to look at your timeline and it will provide you the necessary motivation to keep going. Also, keep a track of your body measurements. At times, you might not notice any weight loss, but you will be able to see a change in your body measurements.

Step 10: Things to keep in mind

If you are getting started with Intermittent Fasting or you want to try this diet, then there are a couple of things that you will need to keep in mind. You need to understand that the initial couple of days might be quite hard. Your body will take some time to get accustomed to the new diet and during this time, you need to fight your urge to give in. You need to stick to this diet for at least three weeks before you can see a visible change in your body. It can difficult to battle your hunger pangs until your body gets used to fasting. So, you need to come up with ways in which you can do so. You will learn more about the different tips that you can follow to make the diet easier in the next chapter.

Follow the simple steps given in this section to devise a plan of action to get started with this diet.

Chapter Nine: Tips and Tricks

Well, now that you know what Intermittent Fasting is all about and the way you can get started, the next step will be to incorporate any of the Intermittent Fasting protocols into your life. In this chapter, let us look at a couple of tips that will come in handy while following the protocols of this diet.

Whenever you feel that a hunger pang is about to strike, take a couple of deep breaths and have a glass of water. The hunger pang must pass you by in less than 15 minutes. If it doesn't ease up, you can have a cup of green tea, herbal tea, or even black coffee.

Whenever you are breaking your fast, don't start gorging on food immediately. You must not try stuffing yourself with as much food as you possibly can but instead, take a couple of minutes and let the intense hunger pass before you start eating. There is no rush, so eat slowly and avoid all sorts of distractions. So, turn the TV off while eating and keep your phone switched off. Don't indulge in mindless eating and practice mindful eating. Enjoy what you are eating and indulge your senses. Don't try to compensate for the fasting period by stuffing yourself with food as you aren't doing yourself any good whatsoever.

It is ideal that you start your meal by having foods that are full of nutrients. So, fill up your plate with food rich in proteins, natural fats, and fiber, instead of carbs and sugars. Protein and fiber will help you feel fuller for longer and will reduce your calorie consumption as well. Nutrition must be your priority and not the quantity of food you consume. If you ever feel like having a cup of ice cream, make sure that you fill yourself up with nutritious food before indulging yourself with a sugary treat.

Try to keep yourself as busy as you possibly can be and don't sit idly. If you are always working, then you won't have any spare time to think about hunger or plan for your next meal. The more you think about food, the hungrier you will feel. Do your best to keep yourself busy.

Your body will take about a week or so to get used to any of the Intermittent Fasting protocols. Once your body is used to it, you can incorporate high-intensity workouts into your exercise schedule. Working out while you are fasting will help to improve the process of weight loss by speeding up the process of burning fats for fuel generation. However, observe caution while doing so. If you feel tired or even fatigued, you must immediately stop what you are doing. Make sure that you always keep your body hydrated.

You might overindulge during an initial couple of days of Intermittent Fasting. At least the first couple of times when this happens, don't panic and don't worry unnecessarily. It is just your body's survival instinct kicking in due to the absence of food. Your survival instinct is hardwired into your brain, and it will take a week or two to condition yourself. After a while, you will start eating regular-sized meals. So, don't worry.

During the eating window, you don't have to count calories and are indeed free to eat anything; however, this doesn't mean that you eat all sorts of junk. You must eat in such a manner that you will not be hungry during your fasting period. If you start feeling hungry immediately after a meal, you can always have a small snack. You must merely make sure that you are sticking to your fasting and feeding schedule.

You must always start out slowly. Remember that neither your body nor your mind is used to not eating for prolonged periods of time. It will take some time to condition yourself. You will be setting yourself up for failure if you think that you can immediately start fasting for 24 hours at a stretch. Instead, work on gradually increasing the gap between two meals. You can also begin by skipping one meal at a time.

You can maintain your blood sugar levels throughout the day by having high-quality carbohydrates like vegetables and fruit along with a lot of protein and naturally fatty food. It will also help your body optimize its ability to burn all the stored fat. Instead of having a meal that's full of carbs, make sure you are getting all the nutrients you need and not just the calories.

You must adjust your eating window in such a manner that your body gets a couple of hours to digest the food you eat before you can sleep at night. Don't go to bed the minute you have finished eating. At times, you might feel slightly hungry before you sleep. However, you must just let that hunger pang pass. You will feel quite full in a right way when you wake up in the morning.

Lack of sleep happens to be one of the significant obstructions to losing weight. So, make sure that you get good quality sleep at night. For optimal functioning of your body and brain, you need about 7 hours of undisturbed sleep daily.

At times, you might have to break your fast before the fasting period ends and it is okay. You don't have to beat yourself up for it. Occasionally, you can have a cheat day. However, make sure that neither of these things is a regular occurrence and just happens to be an isolated incident. Don't let it demotivate you and you must certainly not let it stress you out.

Your mind is the most significant hurdle

Implementing Intermittent Fasting is easy. When you eat depends on the form of Intermittent Fasting you decide to follow. If you want to fast daily, then it can be something as simple as giving your breakfast a miss when you wake up. Instead, you start your eating window with lunch and go about your day as usual. However, there is a mental barrier that you might come across. You might wonder how you can go through your day without breakfast. Do you feel that you will faint if you don't eat or that you will not be able to think straight? These questions are natural, and it is okay if you have any reservations about this diet. When you try this diet, you will understand that all these fears are unwarranted. Nothing will happen to your body if you don't eat one meal a day. In fact, you will feel better and more energetic than you ever did. If you keep thinking that you need to eat every couple of hours or have five meals daily or have your breakfast, or whatever it is that you have convinced yourself of, it is all in your mind. You believe all this because you were told it, not because you ever tried it for yourself. Your ability to think is essential. If you can think differently, you can act differently as well.

It is easy to lose weight

When you tend to eat less frequently, your overall food intake reduces. As a result of all this, you will end up losing weight while you follow Intermittent Fasting. You might plan for big meals but eating them consistently will not be easy. Intermittent Fasting is an excellent idea for all those who want to lose weight because it merely reduces your overall carb intake. Even if you have two large meals daily, the calories you eat will undoubtedly be less than when you ate six meals a day. By merely cutting down on how much you eat, you can lose weight. After all, it is quite simple to lose weight. So, if weight loss is your primary aim, then you accomplish it with this simple diet.

If you want, you can build muscle

You can build muscle while you fast. You don't have to worry about losing muscle while on this diet. Also, the muscle you gain will be lean muscle. If you want a lean and toned body, then this is the best diet for you.

You can work while you fast

You will realize that you are more productive while you're on a fast. Your energy levels will be quite high when you wake up in the morning. The first three hours of the morning will be the most productive portion of the day for you. Well, that's about 12 to 15 hours into your diet, and that's when your body functions optimally. You might believe that your brain will not function optimally when it doesn't get necessary glucose. Well, all that's just a misconception. Since you no longer need to worry about what you can eat for breakfast, you can use this time to do something that's more productive. Your body produces energy while you sleep, and you can utilize this store of power as soon as you wake up. If you want to become productive, then you certainly must give this diet a go.

Cycle what you eat

Intermittent Fasting works well. However, you can make it more efficient by calorie and carb cycling. Do you know what these terms mean? You must have a couple of extra calories on the day you decide to exercise. So, you cycle calories by increasing your food intake. On the other days, you must aim for a calorie deficit. The idea behind this logic is quite simple. You can train to build muscle on all those days you exercise and, on the other days, you can encourage your body to burn fat. You must cycle your carbs on the day you train. It helps to stimulate the loss of fat. Have high protein and low-fat meals on regular days and the days you work out, have some carbs.

It is a lifestyle

We often tend to think of our diets as short-term regimes. It is better to be mindful of what you eat throughout the week instead of just a day or a couple of hours. Whether you have a protein shake 30 minutes before you work out isn't much of an issue if you have a high protein meal within 24-hours of your workout. Intermittent Fasting works because of the eating restriction it places on you. Let us say that you have three meals daily; it is a grand total of 21 meals in a week. Over the course of the diet, do you think your body cares if you eat from 8 a.m. to 8 p.m. in the day or from 1 p.m. to 1 a.m.? How about we stretch it out for a month? Would it make sense to have 80 well-balanced meals so that your body can make the most of it regardless of the time frame within which you eat? It is essential to understand that the food you eat usually has a great impact on your overall health. The diet will not make any sense if you starve yourself daily and then break your fast with all sorts of junk. It is better to think of Intermittent Fasting as a lifestyle choice instead of a mere diet. Not only does it make the diet more practical to follow, but you can maintain your weight loss as well. If you follow the diet religiously for two months and then go back to your unhealthy ways, it will not do your body any good. In fact, all the good that the diet did will be nullified.

You will want less food

When you fast, you will realize that your body craves less food. The diet doesn't victimize you. In fact, it teaches you to listen to your body. You will do what your body tells you to. While you fast, you might think of a hundred different things you want to eat, but when you break your fast, your opinion is bound to change. Once you get used to the diet, you will want to eat only when you are hungry. In a way, Intermittent Fasting curbs mindless eating.

Lose fat and gain muscle

If you want to lose fat and build lean muscle, then you must follow Intermittent Fasting, carb cycling and calorie cycling. It is not practically possible to lose gain muscle and even lose fat simultaneously. To lose weight, your body needs to burn more calories than you consume. So, it is essential to maintain a net calorie deficit to shed weight. However, if you want to build muscle, you need to consume more calories than you burn. It is apparent that you cannot have a net surplus and a net deficit simultaneously. For instance, you can either eat more than 2000 calories or less than 2000 calories at a given point in time. It is the reason why it is impossible to burn excess fat and gain muscle at the same time. However, if you don't think about the small timeframe and think about the diet over the course of a month instead of a day, you have more options available. For instance, you can decide to work out three days in a week, and you can maintain a calorie deficit on all the other days of the week. Therefore, your body will lose fat on a couple of days and gain muscle on the rest. But you cannot do both at the same time. So, you must think about your diet from a long-term perspective instead of a day-to-day diet.

More gains when you fast

There is a simple hypothesis for strength training, and it goes as follows "Always do the most important thing before the rest." It is about prioritizing. It works well not just for your diet, but with any other aspect of your life as well. It is quite simple. You must set one goal for your workout schedule, and you must do the exercises that are more important than others. For instance, let us assume that you work out three days in a week - Monday, Wednesday and Friday. You can do two sessions every session, the upper body workout and the lower body workout. The results you derive from exercise are more when you are fasting.

Fasted state

If you don't exceed 50 calories, your body will stay in a fasted state. There is no scientific evidence about whether it is true or not, but it seems to work for the majority. So, if you like to start your day with a glass of orange juice or a cup of coffee, then you can do so without any worry. Just make sure that your calorie intake doesn't exceed 50 calories. The idea of an intermittent fast is to switch your body to a fasted state instead of a fed state. It is quite easy, and you don't have to make any drastic changes to your daily schedule.

Drink lots of water

You must prepare yourself to drink plenty of water while you fast. Most of us aren't used to drinking a lot of water. In fact, we tend to forget that our body needs water. You can rectify this situation by drinking water. You must have at least eight glasses of water daily, and Intermittent Fasting will help you. Drinking plenty of water helps to detoxify your body and improves the health of your skin as well.

The best diet

Who would not want the ultimate diet plan? Everyone wants one. However, there is no such thing as a perfect diet. The diet that works well for one person might not work for someone else. Some might prefer the 24-hour method and others might like Leangains. The idea is to follow a diet that works well for you. If you want, you can try the different variations of Intermittent Fasting before you select one method. Your body isn't the same as someone else's, and its metabolism differs as well.

It is essential to stay motivated even when you don't seem to lose any weight while on an intermittent fast. So, you successfully made it through the first week or two of Intermittent Fasting, but you don't notice any weight loss? You will probably not see any fat loss within the first two weeks of the diet. Understand that this is normal and it doesn't mean that the diet isn't working for you. Fat loss starts only after three weeks of the diet. So, you need to keep going even when you feel like it's not working. Or maybe you are in a slump and cannot see the results that you once could. Well, it is important that you don't lose faith in the diet and that you keep going even when you don't want to. All that sounds simple, but how can you stay motivated? In this section, you will learn about a couple of simple steps that you can follow to make sure that you stay motivated and on the right track. If you give up now, all the efforts you put in until now will be for nothing.

While you follow Intermittent Fasting, you will feel quite energetic and sharp when you wake up in the morning. In fact, you will feel more energetic than ever. Your body will start to function optimally. The best part about this diet is that you can do everything like you normally would. Concentrate on how good you felt while on this diet, and it will motivate you. A little bit of self-control and self-discipline can help you stay on track. If you feel that a method isn't working for you, try another method and see is that works. Try different foods. It is a process of trial and error. So, don't give up just yet.

Chapter Ten: Mistakes to Avoid

Now that you are aware of the protocols of Intermittent Fasting and the benefits it offers, you must be quite excited to get started! Before you start this diet, you need to be aware of a couple of common mistakes that you need to avoid. If you avoid the mistakes discussed in this chapter, then you can maximize the benefits you derive from this diet.

Mistake 1: Giving up too soon

Intermittent Fasting might not be easy during the initial weeks. You will need to go for prolonged periods of time without eating. Regardless of the method you opt for, you will need some discipline to ensure that you stick to your diet. During the initial week or two, you will need to combat your hunger pangs if you want this diet to be successful. If you can tough it out for a week or so, you will start to see the positive benefits of this diet. So, don't make the mistake of giving up too soon. Instead, trust the process and the diet and you will see positive results within no time.

Mistake 2: Binge Eating

When you break your fast, you might be tempted to stuff yourself with a lot of food. If you start overloading on calories after fasting for 16 hours, it will negate the benefits of this diet. If you indulge in binge eating whenever you break your fast, this diet will not do you any good. Instead, pace yourself and eat slowly. Your stomach takes about twenty minutes to realize when you are feeling full. So, take your time while eating and don't eat if you aren't hungry.

Mistake 3: Not eating enough

You need to eat until you are full and no more than that. If you don't eat anything at all, then you run the risk of starving yourself. If your body shifts into starvation mode, then you cannot achieve your weight loss and health goals. A lot of people worry that they will undo all that they have achieved while fasting if they eat during the eating window. If you do this, then it will be quite difficult to go through the subsequent spell of fasting. Your body needs food to function optimally. So, if you skip meals unnecessarily or if you don't eat enough food, you are merely hurting yourself.

Mistake 4: Wrong Foods

You need to eat the right foods if you want to lose weight or achieve your fitness goals on this diet. It isn't merely about the calories you consume, but about the quality of nutrition you feed your body. If you fast for 12 hours and then eat a tub of ice cream, it certainly will not do you any good! The way your body metabolizes food is quite different. For instance, if you consume 500-caloires of avocado it will be metabolized quite differently from 500 calories of cookies or chips! Also, if you end up eating junk food after breaking your fast, it is quite likely that you will be hungry within no time at all.

The protocols of Intermittent Fasting dictate that you need to eat a healthy and a well-balanced meal after breaking your fast! Ensure that you consume the necessary macros before you think about indulging in any junk food. Fill yourself up with protein and fiber-rich food, healthy dietary fats and some carbs before you even think about reaching for a chocolate bar.

Mistake 6: Forgetting to drink

You need to consume calorie-free beverages throughout the day to keep your body thoroughly hydrated. If you don't drink plenty of water and stay thirsty for long periods, it can trigger unnecessary hunger pangs. Usually, hunger pangs are a sign that your body is thirsty. Also, if you keep your body hydrated, you will feel satiated while fasting.

Mistake 7: Taking it too far

At times, you might not be able to fast for 16 hours at a stretch and you might want to break your fast earlier than usual. If that's the case, then please do so, but don't make a habit of it. You need to learn to listen to your body. Your body knows what it needs. Intermittent Fasting isn't about numbers. Instead, it is about doing what is good for your body. Don't take it too far and risk burning yourself out.

If you avoid the common mistakes discussed in this chapter, it will be quite easy to stick to Intermittent Fasting.

Chapter Eleven: Intermittent Fasting and Weight Loss

Intermittent Fasting has become quite popular recently and it is an effective way of losing weight as well. This method of eating involves fasting for short periods of time. It helps to optimize the production of hormones that assist in controlling the weight. Fasting helps to reduce your calorie consumption. As mentioned in the previous chapters, there are different methods of Intermittent Fasting. The most popular ones happen to be the 16/8 method, eat-stop-eat method and the 5:2 diet. If you don't overeat during the non-fasting periods, you will be able to lose weight.

The effect of Intermittent Fasting on your hormones

The human body stores energy or calories in the form of body fat. Once you restrict your food intake or when you fast, there are several changes that take place in your body, for making this stored energy accessible. The changes in the activity of the nervous system also lead to changes in several important hormones in the body. When you start fasting, your insulin levels will decrease and it helps to burn fat. The production level of the human growth hormone (HGH) also increases. The norepinephrine that is released by the nervous system helps break down the fat stored in cells into fatty acids that help generate energy. Fasting for short periods of time will facilitate burning of fat. However, fasting for prolonged periods of time can suppress your metabolism. Therefore, Intermittent Fasting is a really good idea.

Helps in reducing calories and losing weight

Intermittent Fasting is effective since it helps reduce your calorie consumption. Regardless of the type of fasting method you opt for, you will need to fast for short periods of time. This will help to reduce your calorie consumption. A study that was published in 2014 showed that Intermittent Fasting over a period of 3-24 weeks could help reduce the body weight by 4-8%. The study also showed that people lost belly fat as well. The benefits offered by Intermittent Fasting aren't just restricted to weight loss. It has several metabolic benefits and it can help prevent a few chronic diseases as well. You needn't count calories on your normal eating days. However, on the fasting days make sure that you don't exceed 500-600 calories per day. Intermittent Fasting can easily help you restrict your calorie intake.

Holding on to muscle while you are dieting

When you start dieting, your body not only starts burning fat, but it starts burning muscle as well. There are several studies that show that Intermittent Fasting will help you burn fat without burning any muscle. In one study, it was discovered that the weight loss on Intermittent Fasting was the same as the weight loss that would have resulted from restricting calories for prolonged periods of time. However, there was hardly any reduction in the muscle mass.

Easier to eat healthy

The simplicity of this diet is one of its main advantages. Instead of eating three meals every day, you get to eat two or maybe three small meals every day. This makes things easier. Not only is this diet easy to follow, but it doesn't take much to stick to it either. You get to lose weight and maintain the weight loss over a long period of time.

There are different ways in which you can lose weight. Intermittent Fasting has become a popular method of fasting in the recent past. This method involves fasting for a short duration of time. Fasting for short periods of time will help people to consume fewer calories, and it also helps them optimize the hormones that regulate weight gain or loss. There are different methods of Intermittent Fasting to choose from, and you can opt for a technique that you feel is best suited for you. As long as you fast carefully and don't exceed your calorie intake or binge on junk food on non-fasting days, you are bound to drop those extra pounds.

Weight Loss

Your body stores away energy or calories in the form of body fat. When you don't consume anything, then your body will change several things within itself to make this stored energy available to it. It is all related to the changes in the activities performed by your central nervous system and also changes in the levels of various essential hormones in your body. When you fast, there are a few things that will change your metabolism such as the level of insulin changes when you fast. When you eat, insulin levels increase and when you fast it decreases. A low level of insulin will help burn away the accumulated fat. During a fast, Human Growth Hormone or HGH will increase, and this helps you to gain muscle and reduce fat. Fat cells are broken down into norepinephrine, and this helps in the burning down of fatty acids to generate energy. Despite the widespread belief that consuming five to six small meals is good, short-term fasting helps burn fat. Some studies suggest that fasting for 48 hours can help boost your metabolism and fasting for more than 48 hours can suppress the same. Short-term fasting can lead to several changes in your body and also the hormones that are produced.

Intermittent Fasting will also help you reduce calorie intake and help you lose weight. The reason for the success of Intermittent Fasting works is it reduces the number of calories that you are consuming. The different protocols that you will have to follow during the fasting periods make sure that you aren't eating more calories than those required by your body. If you follow

Intermittent Fasting for three weeks, you will be able to see a change in your body and will have noticed a significant weight loss as well. With alternate day fasting, you can lose up to one 1.7 pounds every week. Intermittent fasting will also help you lose belly fat and will reduce your circumference. These results are indeed awe-inspiring and show that Intermittent Fasting is an excellent tool for assisting you to lose weight.

The benefits of Intermittent Fasting go well beyond just weight loss. It helps to improve your metabolism and will also help you prevent many chronic diseases while expanding your lifespan. Although you needn't count calories when you are on an Intermittent Fasting diet, overall weight loss usually depends on the reduction in the number of calories consumed. A particular study proves that Intermittent Fasting and continuous calorie restriction display the same results when compared amongst members belonging to similar groups. Intermittent Fasting is indeed a very convenient way of restricting the calories consumed without making any conscious effort of trying to eat less.

As mentioned in the previous chapters, Intermittent Fasting not only helps you lose weight but it will also help you hold on to muscle. One of the most prominent side effects of dieting on your body will be the burning of tissue along with fat. Intermittent Fasting can help you shed weight without any reduction in the muscle mass in your body. On a diet with just calorie restrictions, your body will start breaking down muscle to fuel itself. In calorie restriction diets about 25% of the weight loss was muscle mass, and in Intermittent Fasting diets only 10% of weight loss was associated with muscle mass. One study was conducted where the participants were all asked to consume the same amount of calories, except they had to do this in just one huge meal given to them in the evening. They not only lost body fat but also increased their muscle build up, along with a host of other beneficial changes in their health. However, there are a few limitations to the studies that were conducted, so you will probably take these findings with a pinch of salt. When compared to any standard diet you might have tried, Intermittent Fasting will help you hold onto your muscle mass while burning away all the unnecessary body fat.

If you want to succeed at Intermittent Fasting, then there are certain things that you must keep in mind if you're going to be able to lose weight. You will need to make sure that the food that you are consuming is of good quality and you must try eating whole foods whenever possible. You must not forget how important it is to count calories. Don't try to eat too "normally" on your non-fasting days, not so much that you end up compensating for the calories that you didn't consume on your fasting days. It is essential to be consistent. This rule applies to any weight loss method that you might try. You need to try it for a few weeks at least if you want it to work. It will take your body a while to get accustomed to this new fasting protocol. You need to be consistent with your meal schedule, and over a period, this will become easy.

Most of the Intermittent Fasting rules also recommend that you take up strength training. It is essential if you want to burn your body fat while you are still holding onto your muscle mass. During the initial week or two, you needn't bother counting the calories you consume, but after that, you need to be careful. If you feel like your weight loss has stalled, then you must reconsider your calorie intake. The requisites of Intermittent Fasting are that you eat a healthy diet and maintain a negative calorie count or deficit if you want to lose weight. You also must be consistent in your diet and don't forget to exercise.

Well, you need to remember that, at the end of the day, Intermittent Fasting is just a tool that you can make use of when you are trying to lose weight. The primary reason for this is the reduction in your calorie intake. There are specific definite effects essential hormones have on the body that contribute to the same. Intermittent Fasting might not be for everyone, but it might prove helpful if you try it out. So, try Intermittent Fasting for a few weeks, and you will be able to see the change for yourself.

The best way to lose weight is to lose primarily body fat, and when it comes to doing that, nothing beats the one-two knock out combination of proper diet, which we've already covered with the different Intermittent Fasting protocols, and exercise. Exercising helps you not just burn more calories but also helps maintain a fast metabolism – even develop a faster one, which is the ability to burn calories. In this section, we'll take a look at two ways to exercise for weight loss.

Resistance or Weight Training

One of the most popular misconceptions about this type of exercise, especially for women, is that it will lead to super big muscles that'll make ladies look like Dwayne "The Rock" Johnson or Terry Crews. Nothing can be further from the truth. Guys like them are freaks of nature. Even better, women bodybuilders are even rarer. Whether referring to men or women, only 1% of the population has the potential to grow muscles that are that big. Of course, it requires synthetic drugs like steroids too. Given that your chances of bulking up with muscle via resistance training alone are virtually zero, you can breathe normally now. The good news about weight training is instead of bulking up, it will help you reduce your size and you will become leaner. Resistance training, according to studies, can be more effective in burning body fat compared to cardio. It's because it helps maintain muscle mass – increase it even – and muscle mass is key to proper metabolism. Simply put, less muscle mass means a slower metabolism. But again, this doesn't say you'll have to be as big as the Incredible Hulk, Thor, Superman or Captain America.

Oh – and it helps firm and shape up your favorite body parts like the chest, butt and arms, among other parts. Exercise and Intermittent Fasting will help you sculpt the body you always wished for.

Cardiovascular Training

If weight or resistance training is superior to cardiovascular training, why do you need to incorporate it into your weight loss efforts? For one, just because it's not as good doesn't mean it's worthless and doesn't help. The primary benefit of doing this type of training is that it helps make your heart and lungs stronger and more efficient regarding delivering much-needed blood and oxygen all through your body, which is key to better exercise performance and overall health. Another benefit is that it does help burn body fat, though not as much as resistance or weight training. And lastly, it's much easier to do given all you need is a good pair of running or brisk walking shoes and exercise clothes and you can hit the road for a run or walk, which isn't like weight or resistance training, which requires specialized equipment. While you can do bodyweight training, it's often too difficult for beginners.

You'll have to exercise caution when it comes to doing cardio work because if you do too much, your body will start to consume muscle tissue for energy instead of calories and body fat. And given that muscle mass is key to having proper metabolism, less muscle mass means slower metabolism – and less ability to burn body fat. So how much is too much? More than 45 straight minutes of regular cardio and more than 30 consecutive minutes of high-intensity cardio is too much.

Exercise Intensity and Duration

The thread that runs through both resistance and cardio training, particularly when it comes to optimal weight loss, is intensity. Simply put, it means the amount of effort put in.

There are three intensity levels when it comes to exercising – low, moderate and high. The optimal intensity is moderate.

So how do you find out your current exercise intensity level? The most straightforward and relatively accurate way of doing so is called the talk test. After exercising for a couple of minutes, try talking as you continue exercising. If you can still carry on a very normal conversation with no effort whatsoever, it means you're exercising at low intensity, which means it's too easy to burn any significant amount of calories. If you can barely talk or carry on a conversation normally, huffing and puffing throughout, your intensity is high, i.e., too hard. If you can still carry on with a normal conversation, but with some effort or strain in breathing or talking, that's moderate intensity – the perfect intensity for optimal fat burning. Moderate intensity must be maintained for a specific period. Otherwise, it won't help you burn significant calories for weight loss. Exercise for too long puts you at risk of losing muscle mass and for too short a period, at risk of being unable to burn many calories. The optimal window is between 20 to 45 minutes of moderate intensity exercise.

Follow the simple exercising tips given in this chapter to speed up the process of weight loss.

Chapter Twelve: Intermittent Fasting While Travelling

Up until now, you were introduced to different methods of Intermittent Fasting, its benefits, tips to get started and the like. In this section, you will learn about a couple of reasons why Intermittent Fasting is a good idea while traveling.

Efficiency

Let us assume that your flight lands in Frankfurt from New York, but you need to catch a bus, which will take nine hours to meet your pals in Berlin. You need to collect your luggage from the baggage claim, go through the border security, get your bearings, take a cab to the bus station and eat something along the way. Oh wait, you don't have to worry about the last item on your list since you are fasting. It helps you focus on your travel. If you want to reach your destination without any unnecessary delays, then Intermittent Fasting will come in handy.

Save money

If you fast for at least 14 to 16 hours in a day, it means that you can deduct the expenses for at least one meal. If you do this whenever you are traveling, you can save quite a bit. Not just a meal, but you can even reduce your snacking expenses. On an average, you can save anywhere between $30 and $50 per day. So, if you are traveling for a week, you can save close to $300 on your food expenses.

Energy

If you have a sensitive stomach or are used to following a specific diet when you are home, then trying out new foods can upset your stomach. When you fast, you tend to not only save energy but will feel more alert as well. All this energy that you save, you can use while traveling for sightseeing or any other activities.

Control

Things tend to happen - flights or buses can be late, plans can change and you might not speak the local language. You cannot control all these things, but the one thing that you can control is the way you treat your body. Intermittent Fasting will give you a sense of control that you might not otherwise find in a foreign land. Even if you are a frequent traveler, the local culture, language and people can seem quite overwhelming and tiring. If you are used to Intermittent Fasting, then it will give you a sense of routine and normalcy. If you want to hold onto this sense of control, then you simply need to stick to your dieting protocols even when you travel.

Time

Think about all the time that you spend when you need to get food and eat food. In fact, at times, a major portion of your traveling time goes on eating. There is nothing wrong with this. It certainly is exciting trying new things, but the purpose of traveling isn't merely eating. While following the protocols of this diet, you will realize that you have more time to do other activities. All the time that you spend eating is now freed up and you can do whatever you want. Also, if you are in a rush while getting from one place to the next, then at least you don't have to worry about eating.

Cleanse

Intermittent Fasting gives your body an opportunity to cleanse itself. Your body needs a break from all the traveling and the work that you do. Intermittent Fasting is a method of self-cleanse and it is quite simple. When you don't constantly keep pumping food into your system, your system can start cleaning itself.

Chapter Thirteen: Weight Loss on a Budget

Intermittent Fasting sounds like a proper diet, doesn't it? It is a proper diet without the unnecessary frills that come along with a conventional diet. Well, there is more good news for you. You can lose weight while on a strict budget. So, you can improve your health and achieve your weight loss goals while you stick to a budget. This does sound good, doesn't it? It sounds even better in a world that is overrun with different expensive fad diets that will burn a hole in your pocket. In this section, you will learn about certain tips that you can follow to shed those excess pounds while on a budget.

Water, water, and more water

It is quite important that your body is always thoroughly hydrated. Water not only hydrates your body, clears your skin, flushes out the toxins, but it also makes you feel fuller for longer. You must drink at least eight glasses of water per day. Regardless of the method of Intermittent Fasting you want to follow, you must drink plenty of water. Whenever you feel a hunger pang strike you, calm yourself down and drink a glass of water. You must always carry a water bottle with you. You can add a sprig of mint leaves and a couple of slices of lemon to the water to spruce it up.

Eat slowly

You need to learn to eat slowly. Never be in a rush to stuff yourself and instead concentrate on what you are eating. When you eat slowly, the urge to binge fades away. You need to chew your food thoroughly before you swallow it. If you eat slowly, it helps improve the process of digestion and absorption of food. Learn to savor the flavors of the food, the textures and the smells. Try to be mindful of what you are eating, and you can slow yourself down.

Eat healthily

Intermittent Fasting primarily concentrates on when you eat and not what you eat. It doesn't mean that you are free to eat anything that you please. If you want to lead a healthy life and achieve your weight loss objectives, then you need to eat healthy and wholesome meals. The meals that you eat must provide your body the nourishment it needs.

Cook at home

Try to cook at home as often as you can. If you want to save some money on your food bills, then avoid buying prepacked meals. It might seem quite easy to order a salad, but it will be quite expensive in the long run. You don't need any fancy ingredients while following Intermittent Fasting, so you don't have to buy a lot of groceries. You can cook simple meals and home and ensure that you eat at home. Instead of ordering a $10 salad, you can buy a big bag of mixed salad greens for $5 and have two meals instead of one!

Ration your portions

You must control the portions you eat. You can do this by weighing out the portions you eat. The meals you consume need to be rich in protein and fiber, while low in carbs. If you eat plenty of fiber, protein and the right amount of dietary fats, then your body will obtain all the necessary nutrients that it needs to stay healthy.

Plan your meals

With Intermittent Fasting, you can select your eating window. When you know this, you can easily plan for your meals in advance. If you know that you will be fasting all day long, then make sure that there is a tasty meal waiting for you at home. By doing this, you will effectively reduce the urge to eat out.

Grocery shopping

Grocery shopping might seem like a chore, but it is quite important. Before you decide to head out, you need to make a list of all the groceries that you need. You don't need any junk food or unhealthy foods stored at home if you are trying to eat healthily. So, the first thing that you need to do is clear your pantry off all the food items that aren't healthy. Also, you must never shop when you are hungry.

You must not only prepare a food list, but you need to make sure that you stick to it while shopping. It is quite easy to cook if you have all the necessary ingredients readily available. Shop for your groceries once a week and if you plan your meals in advance, you will know the groceries you need to buy.

Meal prep

You must make it a habit of doing the basic meal prep over the weekends. It helps you prepare for the week that lies ahead. Meal prep is quite simple, and it can something as basic as cutting or chopping up vegetables. You can make a couple of simple curry pastes or stews and freeze them. You can even partially cook meats and freeze them. You can pretty much freeze anything that you want. For instance, you can make a Thai curry paste and freeze it. So, on a weekday, you merely need to add some protein and vegetables to the curry paste and voila, your meal is ready.

One of the best things that you can cook in batches and freeze is broth! You can use the broth to make soups, stews, and curries.

Eat fruit for dessert

If you have a sweet tooth, it might feel challenging to give up on desserts. So, to satiate your sweet cravings, you can have fruit for dessert. A cup of strawberries with a tablespoon of unsweetened whipped cream is a tasty dessert. Have berries or any other fruit that you want. Fruit is good for your body and are full of nutrients. However, you must be mindful of the hidden calories they consist of. You must not have three mangoes just because it is a fruit. Eat healthily! For instance, frozen bananas with some peanut butter, or apple wedges with peanut butter make for a tasty sweet treat. There are plenty of healthy alternatives for desserts and try them out.

Food budget

You must set a weekly or a monthly food budget for yourself. It isn't about merely setting a budget, but you also need to make sure that you stick to the budget. When you are planning your food budget, you need to make sufficient allocations for grocery shopping. It helps you keep a track of your expenses. You can always download a mobile application to track your spending.

Eat the healthy stuff first

Whenever you break your fast, you might be overcome by the urge to eat a lot of food. Your body might start craving for carbs and sugar. So, you need to make sure that you eat all the healthy stuff before you even think about eating anything unhealthy. If you want a scoop of ice cream or a bar of chocolate, you must tell yourself that you can eat that stuff after you eat all the necessary protein and fiber. Once your tummy is full, then the urge to eat will also reduce. If you do this, you will not feel like you are denying yourself anything.

Brush your teeth after eating

It is a healthy habit to brush your teeth before you go to sleep at night. Ensure that you brush your teeth after dinner. In a way, it is a signal to your body that you have finished with the meals for any given day. It certainly helps on a psychological level. Not only will you have stronger and cleaner teeth, but it also reduces the urge to want to eat.

Don't leave the house hungry

You must never leave the house hungry. How often do you purchase a cup of coffee on your way to work? Coffee will certainly wake you up in the morning, but how much do you spend on your morning fix-me up? If you are used to buying coffee daily, then you will spend about $5 in one go. That's about $150 a month and $1800 a year! That's a lot of money that you can use for something else. Instead, why don't you brew your coffee at home and take it along with you? That's not only simple but is quite inexpensive as well.

Also, you must never leave the house hungry. If your fasting period ends and you want to head out for a meal, make sure that you snack on something healthy before heading out.

Make your snacks

You don't have to buy diet snacks anymore. You can make your own 100-calorie snacks at home and carry them with you. It is quite easy to make your own snacks at home. For instance, it doesn't take more than ten minutes to whip up a batch of kale chips or popcorn. You can store them in small containers and eat whenever you are hungry.

Track what you eat

You can maintain a food journal or use one of the food tracking apps to keep tabs on what you eat. The key is to make a list of everything that you eat. It will help you to eat healthily and cut down on any mindless snacking. When you start tracking what you eat, you will automatically become conscious of the things you are feeding your body.

Exercise

You don't need an expensive gym membership to exercise. There are plenty of different ways in which you can exercise without heading to the gym. You can go for a run, jog or even do yoga at home.

We all have incredibly hectic schedules and lead busy lives and at such a time, it might be difficult to follow a diet. Well, you no longer have to worry about this. The tips explained in this chapter will help you follow the protocols of Intermittent Fasting without burning a hole in your pocket.

Chapter Fourteen: Get Lean while Eating Out

Why is Intermittent Fasting so effective? This diet is quite filling. When you skip breakfast and eat at noon, you are giving yourself the necessary room to eat later. Most of us tend to eat a lot of food at night and that's due to a primitive urge present within us. Once you get used to fasting, you will feel quite focused during the morning and will be able to appreciate the food that you eat later. You can do all this while making sure that you are maintaining a calorie deficit.

Another reason for the popularity of this diet is that it is quite simple. In this busy world that we live in, most of us don't have the time to eat five to six perfectly balanced small meals. It just isn't possible. So, the idea of eating two big and filling meals per day fits in with the hectic schedule of our lives. It also offers a certain degree of flexibility that is necessary.

Intermittent Fasting is designed in such a way that it supports your calorie and macronutrient requirements. It means that by following this dieting protocol, it is quite difficult to exceed your calorie intake. The meal plan that you need to follow ensures that you can consume a lot of protein and fiber that makes you feel full and helps you build lean muscle. Because of all this, it is quite easy to meet your weight loss and fitness goals.

In this section, you will learn about a couple of different strategies that you can follow while eating out.

Strategy 1: Nutrition plan

The first thing that you need to do is track your nutritional intake while at home and you must be aware of the number of calories that you consume, the size of the portions and the composition of your meals. For instance, if you consume 1800 calories in three meals, your dinner can make up for 700 calories, lunch for 400 calories and the rest for another meal. It means that you can have about 70g of protein for lunch and dinner and about 40g in another meal.

Strategy 2: Stick to the Same Foods

Once you establish your calculated nutrition plan, it is all about sticking to it as much as you can while eating out. Ideally, you must try to stick to similar foods to those that you eat while at home. For instance, if you are used to a meal of meats and vegetables, then order something similar when you go out for a meal. If you go out for a meal, stick to the protein and fibers you eat at home and skip any carb and sugar-rich foods.

Strategy 3: Increase Protein

If you aren't sure what to eat and cannot decide, a simple thing that you can do is to increase the portion of the protein you order. You can double up the protein and it will help make you feel full. It isn't just about picking a protein, but you need to pick the protein wisely. It doesn't make any sense if you binge on fried chicken or ribs slathered in barbeque sauce. Avoid all the high-calorie options on the menu. Instead, you must opt for leaner meats like lamb, steak, chicken or fish.

Strategy 4: Carbs

You need to be careful about the amount of carbs you consume. If the dish you ordered has more carbohydrates than you are used to consuming, then simply skip the carbs. You need to avoid carbs as much as possible if you want to speed up the process of weight loss. Carbs will fill you up for a while and then you will feel hungry again. Instead, fill up on the foods that are good for you. If there is a breadbasket on the table, please resist the urge of reaching for it.

Strategy 5: Post Meal Hunger

If you want to have a dessert or still have the urge to eat more, even though you are aware that it will exceed your ideal calorie intake, then you need to know that this feeling of hunger will subside soon. A simple trick is to have a cup of tea after a meal and it will make you feel full. You can also go for a walk after eating and you will feel full. It takes about 20 minutes for your brain to signal to you that you are full so don't keep stuffing yourself with food.

If you follow these simple steps, you can stick to your diet even when you go out for a meal.

Chapter Fifteen: How to set up a Plan (i.e. 8-Week Meal Plan)

Let's get started with making a plan for your Intermittent Fasting. A good plan will be your guide on what you should do and how you should maintain your diet. There are a few steps to creating the perfect plan for your body.

First choose the fasting method that you think you can work with. Decide the duration and frequency that you want to fast for.

Think of your eating habits in general and choose from the type of Intermittent Fasting that will suit you. If one type doesn't suit you, just change and try another. There is no harm in trying out what works best for you in the long run.

You need to notice your usual eating habits and decide which type of eating personality you have. Generally, there are three eating personalities amongst people; Type A, Type B and Type C. Use the following information to find out which type applies to you.

- Type A: Consider yourself lucky if you have Type A eating personality. This type of eating makes fasting easy for you. You will find Intermittent Fasting surprisingly simple for you to follow and stick to. Normally if you unintentionally don't eat for long period of time, this is your personality type. It is not the same as intentionally starving yourself so keep that in mind. You are usually the type who gets busy with other things and tends to forget meals until hunger really strikes. Type A people generally don't tend to try any random diets and fasting might be a first for them. You also don't feel anxious and compulsive about food. If all of this is true for you, you now know your eating personality type.

- Type B: People with this eating personality like to make sure that they eat all their meals on time. It is usually embedded in your mind that you need to eat every single proper meal and get anxious if you miss any. You also are not comfortable about going on any diets and don't do well when you try a diet. Type B personalities always try to make up for skipped meals even when they aren't hungry.
- Type C: Intermittent Fasting is usually the most difficult for people with the tendencies of Type C. However, this is the type that tends to try out diets the most and usually fails. You might be binge eating and have cravings all the time. Type C also don't like missing any meals and eat to make up for any skipped meals. You get anxious and think too much about when and what you will eat. This type of eating personality generally tends to overeat and has weight issues over time.

However, Intermittent Fasting will work for you no matter which type of eating personality you have. It just helps you to define what your eating habits are and how you should try this type of fast. For Type C eating personality, it is recommended to go slow and try your best to stick to the plan but without stressing out about any missed days. The other two types can usually start out with at least 2 days of fasting a week even from their first day. No matter what your type is, just make a plan that you are comfortable with and motivate yourself to stick to it in order to reach your end goal.

A Type A eating personality makes it easy for you to start any fasting diet plan right away. You will see that it is not too different from your usual habits but don't overdo it. Set memos that will remind you to eat on time. Starving yourself for too long will do more harm than good. Try two days of 20-hour fasts on the first week and add another day to this the second week.

Type B eating personality people should go a little slower than Type A. Slowly build up the pace of your fasting without stressing too much about it. Getting anxious about food is not healthy. You can start with 18-20 hour fasts on the first week and do the same the second week but try to add a couple of hours to it.

Type C eating personality people need to be more cautious about their fasting. You need to take it at a slow pace so that it does not overwhelm you but also make sure that you don't give up too soon. You have to build a plan that you know you can stick to. Don't set unrealistic goals or expect too much from yourself. If you try to fast the same as Type A and B people you will actually trigger binge eating quite soon into your plan. Instead take it a day at a time.

On days that you feel you can't, just let it go but adjust it the next day. Set goals for every week. For the first week try an 18-hour fast for one day. Enjoy your normal eating on the other days but be a little conscious about trying to compensate for the day you fasted or will fast again. Don't eat too much just when you break your fast. The next week make it an 18-hour fast on 2 days of the week with at least two days of rest in between these. Fasting for too long will make you sick. Try to be determined for the course of the fasting that you decide on.

Decide on the day that you want to start your fasting. Once you decide, don't budge on it and begin on that very day. Keep some drinks that are non-calorific around. Remember to stay hydrated even if you aren't eating. Water is essential for your body. Keep a timer on your phone to mark the end of your fast. This way you can expect a notification for when you can eat again.

If you are a Type A personality for eating, then begin with an 18-hour fast in your first week and then a 24-hour fast. If you want to try at least 15-hour fasts on a daily basis, keep these on alternate days for your first week of fasting.

If you are a Type B personality for eating then try a 16-hour fast after dinner on your first week. Let it last until lunchtime the next day. Then try to increase a couple of hours and try again after a few days. The next week you can try to make it a 24-hour fast.

For Type C personalities, try a 16-hour fast from evening until 10 a.m. the next day on your first week. Then try again the next week and try to do this twice in a week. Let it build up as you go from there.

Take some notes during your fasting for the first two times. Write down how you felt both physically and mentally. If you feel sick or nauseous at any point, we recommend consulting the doctor.

Let's take a look at a sample plan to get started. This particular plan is more suitable for anyone who just wants to get a head start on Intermittent Fasting and wants to continue it as a part of their lifestyle.

Week One

Let's assume you start fasting on a Sunday. Begin after dinner around 7 p.m. Then keep fasting until 1 p.m. on Monday. Don't fast on this Tuesday and eat like you normally would. Keep your Wednesday fast free as well. On Thursday start fasting after lunch around 1 p.m. and fast until lunchtime on Friday. Do not fast on this next Saturday and Sunday. If the first day was too hard for you, just keep it as one day of fasting for the first week.

When you begin, you need to remember to pace your body. Don't ever fast for two days in a row. Keep a gap of at least two days between each fast. If the hours were too long for your first few days, just reduce a couple and adjust according to your capacity. You can build it up over the next few weeks. The goal is to focus long-term benefits and not short-term failures.

Week Two'

For this second week, keep your first week experience in mind. Decide on the hours that you think will suit you this week and try to increase it even if for one hour. Make the fasting fit around your lifestyle. Choose the days that would suit you and your work and commitments. We are just giving you a sample that you can work with.

This Sunday start fasting after dinner around 9 p.m. and fast until 7 p.m. on Monday. Try to implement a 24-hour fast for this second week if you feel up to it. Don't fast for Tuesday or Wednesday. Eat lunch and start fasting around 1 p.m. on Thursday and break the fast at 1 p.m. on Friday. Don't fast any more for your second week. Don't overeat after your fast is over. This means that you fast for 2 days on your second week.

Week Three

If week two went as planned, you can adjust and increase your times for week three. Start fasting after dinner on Sunday around 9 p.m. Then break the fast around 1 p.m. on Monday. Eat healthy meals for this next two days. On Wednesday, start fasting after lunch around 3 p.m. and break it on Thursday for breakfast around 10am. The next fast should be for half a day from Friday night after dinner at 9 p.m. to 9 a.m. the next day. This just gives you a few extra hours this week to fast.

Week Four

This week try fasting for a few days in shorter intervals. Begin your fast at 8 p.m. on Sunday night and break it by 1 p.m. on Monday. Then fast from 8 p.m. on Tuesday until 1 p.m. on Wednesday and fast again from Thursday from 8 p.m. to Friday until 1 p.m. These will help give you another kind of pace.

Week Five

This week you can start trying to fast every day for 16-18 hours other than the weekend. Eat like you normally do until Sunday dinner and fast from 8 p.m. until 12 p.m. on Monday. Until Friday you have to fast every day and you are allowed to eat only from 12 p.m. to 7 p.m. each day. The 18 hours in between each day's intervals will be for fasting. On Saturday and Sunday give yourself a break. If you couldn't do every single day, take a break in between and don't feel guilty.

Week Six

See how week five went for you. Were you able to try the fast on all the weekdays? You actually get to eat both lunch and dinner for this. If it did not work and you took some days off, try the same routine as week five for week six. Give your body and mind another chance to tough it out.

Week Seven

I'm sure you have the hang of it by now. You can see how it gets easier over time. Try fasting on every alternate day this week. Don't let your body get used to one particular routine. This way you won't have to lead a very strict schedule. Fast from Sunday 7 p.m. to Monday 12 p.m. don't fast until Tuesday 8 p.m. again and repeat these steps for every other day. This week will be much easier. Try to get some exercise in when you are not fasting. Exercising on fasting days will be too taxing for your body.

Week Eight

This is the last week for your set plan. If you have been eating healthy and following the fasting plan, you have already seen changes. It should now be much easier to fast for hours at a time. Week Seven was a break so fast a little extra for this final week.

Start fasting on Sunday at 8 p.m. and eat at 1 p.m. on Monday. Then fast from Monday 8 p.m. until 5 p.m. on Tuesday. Start a fast at 1 p.m. after lunch on Wednesday and break it at dinner on that day. Don't fast on Thursday and then fast from Thursday 8 p.m. until 5 p.m. on Friday. Take a break from fasting now.

You will notice how each week, it gets much easier to follow a plan. The plan helps you mark out what times you can eat and when you can't. It helps you avoid binge eating and reaching for snacks without considering the time. You can eat normally when you are not fasting. But remember not to overeat the meal right after you break your fast. Give your body time to adjust. Also, don't think that you can reward yourself too much after a fast. You should still try to watch what you are eating during your eating intervals. If you load up on too many carbs during your meals, your weight will not show much change. These first few weeks are important to create a healthier lifestyle for yourself. Use the schedule to discipline yourself. There is still a lot of room for adjustment as you go from week one to eight. After you finish week eight, you can decide what type of Intermittent Fasting works best for you. Try to make a plan every month on how you want to keep implementing fasting in your habits. Mark down the events and occasions that you want to enjoy with your family or friends eating good food. It's a good idea to fast on the day after such events. Hydrate yourself with water and herbal teas during your fast. Avoid overeating whether you are at home or away from home. Overeating encourages a type of compulsive eating that you need to learn to grow out of. The Intermittent Fasting helps curb such habits when you know you aren't supposed to touch food during specific hours. So, don't undo all your hard work in a moment of weakness. Learn from the experience.

After your eight weeks, you will see how your body looks and feels differently. Healthier eating always has a good impact on the body. You have probably been drinking a lot of water as well and this can make the appearance of your skin much better. If your want proof of the health benefits, why not go to a doctor before and after these eight weeks of planned Intermittent Fasting? They can help to show you the difference it has made. Your energy levels will be much higher than when you used to overeat every single day. Don't live to eat, eat to live but you can still enjoy the foods you love. Let your food and habits improve the state of your mind and body. Fasting allows your body time to actually use up the reserved energy and food you have consumed. It also makes you feel more conscious of everything you do and you will see improvements all around.

Give it a chance and follow the fasting timings that are given above. It allows you to slowly make fasting a part of your life without burdening you like other diets. You don't have to throw out your favorite chocolates and stop eating your cookies. You just have to learn to eat as much as your body actually needs and not too often.

Chapter Sixteen: Keeping Up the Motivation

Now that you know all about Intermittent Fasting, you've probably tried it for at least a week or two. But are you frustrated because you aren't seeing any visible results? Do you feel like you haven't lost any weight? Or even worse, do you feel like you have gained some?

Intermittent Fasting is not like other fad diets that assure you of weight loss in a few days. You won't see quick results that will make you want to keep doing it until you reach your goal weight. It is a diet that needs patience and will show you results in time according to your body. You need to let your body lose weight in a healthy way and not by trying to rush it. Even if you feel negative because of the rise in the weight scale, there are a few normal reasons for it. Give it time and you will see the opposite happen in a few weeks. Consistency is key to anything. If you don't persist in going through the diet properly, you can't expect to see results.

Let's look at how you can keep yourself motivated in the long run. Start focusing on what's going right in your life and not what's wrong with it. This diet is just a part of it. Just starting with the diet means that you are taking a step in the right direction. Focus on going through all your regular activities and work that needs to be done. Get those completed and stay patient with your fasting diet. In fact, fasting actually gives you more time to focus on other things. The end of the fast has a different effect on your body and you will feel it.

Intermittent Fasting also helps to build your self-discipline and self-control. Every day that you fast allows you to see how far you can go and control your usual instincts. Reaching out for snacks or any food is quite instinctive and that is why people gain a lot of weight. You, on the other hand, know what's right and are trying to keep your body healthy. Even if you have cravings in the middle of the day, you are still suppressing them and make it through to the night. You need to remind yourself and appreciate that you are doing your best every day. Going through each day until the end of your diet plan is what will help you see weight loss and a better body.

When you can't depend on yourself or feel like you aren't sure of the diet, look for inspiration in others. There are lots of other people who have tried the Intermittent Fasting diet and have watched it work for them. There are books, articles, YouTube videos, etc. that are proof of their successful results. People who struggle with weight loss often share their journey. When you see their stories, you will realize that instant gratification is not the way to a fit body. You need to have control over your diet and habits. That is the only way you can achieve the goal you set for yourself.

There are many benefits that you can reap from Intermittent Fasting other than weight loss. It has been shown to help detoxify your body, regulate blood sugar levels, improve brain health, etc. It is not just about losing weight. You need to lose some unwanted fat and gain muscle. This might be the same weight on the scale but it will produce a different and better body shape. The same number will still show changes in the measurements of your body. You will feel and look a lot different over time and this is the healthy change you need to aim for. So, don't lose hope too soon.

You have to remember that weight loss is a journey that will give you bad days and good days. You need to stay strong and determined if you want the Intermittent Fasting to work for you. Try to enjoy the process and you will reap the fruits of your hard work.

Chapter Seventeen: How to Keep the Weight Stable

If your main goal with Intermittent Fasting is to lose weight, you need to keep some things in mind. Weight loss is a process and after that you need to still balance your habits to keep in good shape. If you follow the diet right and work with it, you will definitely see the weight loss in a few weeks. However, your goal should be long-term fitness and health benefits. If you think you can get back to your old habits right after the diet is over, you're wrong. You can eat what you want during and after the diet but it is important to keep your self-control. You learn how to control unhealthy eating with the help of Intermittent Fasting. This is something your mind and body will remember even after your 8-week plan is over. So, utilize your new habits and exercise the self-control needed to stay in good health.

Don't make things too hard on yourself. Unlike other diets, this diet allows you to be flexible. If you have a dinner planned with your friends on a fasting day, just go for it. You can still make up for it later. The point is not to eat too much unnecessarily every single day. Fasting after a night out will help you detoxify if you make it a habit once in a while. If you want to make a plan for yourself, keep any family events in mind and mark other days for fasting. This way you won't miss out on what you want and if you do, you will just be more likely to give up the diet altogether at some point. Be kind to yourself, changes take time.

Don't be extreme in trying to lose weight. Learn to love your body and try to include healthy habits to show it the care it deserves. Stay away from any fad diets that tell you to stop eating for a week or to just drink juices. These will never help you in the long term and can actually harm your body. Eat the food you love from time to time so that you can avoid binge eating. Forbidden things are always a temptation. Instead of overdoing it, just eat a little once in a while so that you don't think about it or have any unhealthy cravings on your fasting days.

Be realistic about your diet and expectations. Also try to add some sort of physical exercise every single day. Even if you just go for a walk, it counts for something. It is not necessary to hit the gym every day like a fanatic but if you like it, then it will definitely speed up the process. Exercise keeps your system running well and your body fit. If you like waking up early then why not try a run around the park. One of the best ways to keep yourself motivated is to do this with a friend. You won't get bored and you can depend on someone to check up on you once in a while. Make it as easy for yourself as possible. You don't have to exert yourself beyond your limits. Don't believe anyone who tries to tell you that you have to hit the gym twice a day to get the body you want. In fact, too much exercise can actually harm you. Just think of it as a simple activity you can inculcate in your routine a few times a week to keep your blood pumping.

Chapter Eighteen: Busting Intermittent Fasting Myths

Intermittent Fasting has immense benefits. Although the concept of going without food for longer periods may seem dreadful to many, fasting has time and again proved to be greatly beneficial for human health. Not eating for longer periods is not only therapeutic for the body, but also boosts a person's immune system, enhances person's insulin sensitivity, recycles old damaged cells, improved DNA repair and offers protection against many other disease. But the most talked about benefits of Intermittent Fasting is weight loss.

The increasing popularity of Intermittent Fasting has also given rise to some myths. Below, we are going to bust some of the most common myths about snacking, fasting and meal frequency.

Skipping breakfast makes you fat

For years, we have been fed this belief that "Breakfast is the most important meal of the day." How many of us question the authenticity of this question? I bet not many. Most people believe that skipping breakfast can result in cravings, hunger and even weight gain in some cases. While a lot of observational researchers have found statistical links between obesity and skipping breakfast, it could be that the quintessential breakfast skipper may not be a health-conscious person overall. A study was published in 2014 that compared people who ate breakfast versus people who skipped breakfast. The 16-week study concluded that there was no significant weight loss difference between the two groups. That said, there have been certain studies, which show that teenagers and children might benefit from eating breakfast by performing better at school. Eating breakfast could be beneficial for some people while for others it might not be as beneficial.

Increase in the frequency of meals helps to boost your metabolism

A lot of nutritionists believe that eating small meals throughout the day can help to accelerate your metabolism. It's certainly true that the human body can expand some amount of energy by assimilating and digesting the nutrients in a meal. This phenomenon is known as the thermic food effect (TEF) which adds up to 30% calories for protein, between 0-3 % for fats and 5-10% for carbohydrates. Overall, the impact of the thermic food is about 10% of a person's total calorie intake. Here, what actually matters is not the amount of meals you consume, but the actual calories that were consumed.

When you eat seven 400-calorie meals in a day, it has a similar effect as eating three 700-calorie meals a day. If you measure the thermic effect here, of 10%, it amounts to 210 calorie in both cases. This fact has also been supported by several feeding studies conducted on humans which show that the increase of decrease in meal frequency is not associated or has no impact on the total calories burned.

Eating frequently prevents you from over eating and reduces hunger

Some of us believe that frequent snacking can help reduce cravings or prevent hunger. When you look at some of the studies conducted on this belief, there has been an interesting mix of evidence. While some studies have shown that an increased frequency in meals results in reduced hunger, others show an increased level of hunger. A particular study that compared 6 high protein meals and 3 high protein meals, it was found that the 3 high-protein meals were more effective in reducing hunger in the participants. However, such an impact could totally vary from person to person. If you feel that snacking helps you stay away from cravings or reduces the chances of you binging, then go for it no matter what the studies say.

There has been no scientific evidence that snacking often or consuming frequent meals can guarantee reduction in your hunger pangs. You can choose what works for you.

Smaller meals can help you lose weight

There has been no evidence that smaller meals boost your metabolism. They also do not contribute toward reducing your hunger pangs. If you consider the fact that consuming frequent meals has no impact on the energy balance equation, then technically it won't have any impact on weight loss either. This fact was also supported scientifically. Several studies that were conducted on his topic showed that meal frequency has no impact on weight loss.

For instance, a research that was conducted involving 16 obese males and females showed that none of the participants experienced any difference in fat loss, weight or appetite when comparing 6 or 3 meals each day.

That said - you might find that eating smaller meals more frequently can make it easier for you to control your cravings, then this could be effective for you. It's also possible that if you have digestion issues, then you can benefit from breaking down your meals in smaller meals. In general, I find it difficult to eat so often which makes it harder for me to control my diet. But it may work for some people.

Your brain requires a constant supply of glucose

We have always believed that eating carbs every few hours is the only way to keep our brains functioning well. This belief could be rooted in the fact that our brains use only glucose as a source of fuel. However, what we don't discuss is that our body is capable of easily producing glucose it requires via a process called gluconeogenesis. Now, this is not required in all cases as your body is already used to storing glycogen in the liver. These glycogen stores can be used to provide enough energy for the brain for hours.

The same goes for long-term fasting. Even when you fast for longer hours, consume a low-carbohydrate diet or starve, your body can produce ketones from dietary fats. Ketone bodies are known for offering energy for most part of the brain while being able to reduce its glucose requirement completely. So, when a person fasts, his or her brain is easily able to sustain by using the ketones as well as the glucose that is produced from fats and proteins.

If you look at it form an evolutionary perspective, the belief that humans wouldn't be able to survive without a consistent supply of carbohydrates is completely senseless. If this fact were true, then the human species would have become extinct a long time ago.

That said - some people might feel hypoglycemic if they go longer periods without eating anything. If you have had the same experience, then you should consume more and more meals throughout the day. But before you make any dietary changes, do consult your doctor and ask for his suggestions regarding this dietary approach.

Snacking and eating frequently is good for health

It is unnatural for the body to stay in a constantly fed state. Back in the day when humans were still evolving, they had to experience food scarcity quite frequently. Scientifically, there has been some evidence suggesting that short-term fasting can trigger a cellular repair phase called autophagy. What is autophagy? It's a process where the human cells make use of dysfunctional and old proteins for energy.

Autophagy is known to help protect humans from developing diseases such as Alzheimer's disease, cancer or even help reduce signs of aging. The fact is that fasting has time and again proved to be beneficial for our metabolic health. Some studies have shown that eating often and snacking can in fact have a negative impact on human health.

For instance, one particular research has shown that frequent meals along with a high calorie intake can result in increased liver fat, implying that snacking often can increase the risk of developing fatty liver disease. Some observations studies have also proved that people who snack often or eat frequent meals are at a higher risk of developing colorectal cancer.

Fasting puts your body in starvation mode

This is one of the most common myths against Intermittent Fasting. A lot of people seem to believe that Intermittent Fasting can put you in starvation mode. As per a lot of claims, when you don't eat, your body thinks that it is starving, so it starts shutting down the metabolism which further hinders you from burning fat. Long-term weight loss can certainly cause a reduction in the amount of calories you burn and put you in starvation mode. This impact can cause less calories to be burned each day.

However, this effect takes place with weight loss regardless of the technique you use. There has been no evidence showing that this only happens when you are fasting or that it doesn't happen with other weight loss methods. So, it's a bit unfair to single out Intermittent Fasting. In fact, there has been some evidence that shows short-term fasts can result in an increase in metabolic rate. This generally happens due to a spike in norepinephrine content in the blood which causes break down of body fat while stimulating a person's metabolism.

Several studies have shown that when you fast up to 48 hours, your metabolism gets a boost of 3.6-14%. But when someone fasts longer than that then the chances are the impact can reverse, causing the metabolism to go down as compared to the baseline.

Your body is capable of using only a certain amount of protein for each meal

This is another topic that has been debated over the years. There are some people who claim that humans are only capable of digesting 30 grams of protein per meal. They also suggest that eating every 2 or 3 hours can help maximize muscle gain. That said - this theory is not supported by science. Studies do not have any evidence that there is a difference in muscle mass of a person if she or he consumes protein in smaller doses. Time and again, it has been proved that it's the total amount of protein consumed by us matters and not the amount of meals it's spread over.

Fasting can make you lose muscle

The common belief is that fasting can make our bodies lose muscle and start using it as fuel. While there's some truth to this phenomenon when people diet in general, there has been no specific evidence that it occurs more with fasting as compared to other weight loss methods. In fact, there have been certain studies which suggest that fasting can actually be largely beneficial for maintaining muscle mass.

In a particular study, intermittent calorie restriction resulted in the same amount of weight loss like calorie restriction. However, there was less reduction in muscle mass. Another study was conducted involving participants who consumed the same amount of calories as before only exception of one big meal in the evening. These participants lost a lot of body fat while having a modest amount of increase in their muscle mass. They also experienced a lot of other health benefits due to fasting.

Intermittent Fasting is also extremely popular particularly among bodybuilders who found it to be effective in maintaining high amounts of muscle while having a low body fat percentage.

Fasting is bad for our health

A lot of people assume that fasting does more harm to the body than good. But this couldn't be further from the truth. Several studies have shown that Intermittent Fasting as well as intermittent calorie restriction can offer impressive health benefits. For instance, Intermittent Fasting can cause the expression of genes linked with longevity to undergo a change and has proven to prolong lifespan in animals. Fasting also offers a lot of benefits for our metabolic health, which includes reduction in oxidative stress, insulin sensitivity, and reduction in the possibility of heart disease.

It has also been found that fasting can actually benefit our brain health by boosting a hormone known as rain-derived neurotropic factor (BDNF). This can be used to protect us against depression as well as other brain-related issues.

Intermittent Fasting makes us overeat

There are some claims that suggest that Intermittent Fasting, instead of causing weight loss, makes us lose weight, as fasting tends to make you overeat during the eating periods. This is true, but only in part. In short, people only end up compensating for the calories that are lost during fasting by consuming more food during the eating window.

That said, this compensation isn't absolute. One particular study has shown that participants who fasted for an entire day ended up consuming an additional 500 calories the next day. These participants expended 2400 calories approximately during the fasting period and ended up overeating by 500 calories the day after. If you so the math, the total reduction in their calorie intake was about 1900 calories and this is a huge deficit considering it's only for 2 days.

The truth is that Intermittent Fasting is one of the most effective tools to lose weight. Stating that starvation can make you overeat and gain weight is completely untrue.

Conclusion

I want to thank you once again for purchasing this book and I hope you enjoyed it.

Intermittent Fasting is a great diet, isn't it? Fasting for extended periods can help achieve your weight loss goals while improving your overall health. Intermittent Fasting is a flexible diet and you can customize it according to your lifestyle needs and convenience.

There are multiple benefits this diet offers. Select a fasting protocol that you can easily incorporate into your daily schedule. If you can add a little exercise to your schedule, you can even build lean muscle! So, all that you need to do now is get started as soon as possible!

Finally, if you enjoyed this book, then I'd like to ask you for a favor, would you be kind enough to leave a review for this book on Amazon? It'd be greatly appreciated!

Thank you and good luck!

Resources

https://anthonymychal.com/intermittent-fasting-mistakes/

https://www.dietdoctor.com/intermittent-fasting

https://dailyburn.com/life/health/intermittent-fasting-exercise-weight-loss/

https://www.healthline.com/nutrition/10-health-benefits-of-intermittent-fasting

http://romanfitnesssystems.com/articles/intermittent-fasting-faq/

https://www.healthline.com/nutrition/11-myths-fasting-and-meal-frequency#section8

Preview of Keto Diet: The Beginners Guide For Men And Women With Ketogenic Diet

The Keto Diet is the new trend in smart eating to lose weight – the reason why it has been able to capture such attention is because of its unique approach. The Keto Diet is all about eating high contents of fat and low contents of carb. When people first hear this they're always surprised because how can eating more fat make us slimmer? Well, that's because fats have been heavily stigmatized which is why all of us believe that it's only fats that make us fat when actually it's the carbs and sugars that we consume every day.

There are fats that are terrible for your body and you should avoid them, but there are also some good fats that help your body to absorb more vitamins and minerals from the food you consume. A high-fat diet doesn't just help you to lose weight, but also improves your cognitive abilities, cholesterol and even provides safety against many diseases.

The purpose of a keto is to make your eating habits a little more natural so that you stop consuming food that is artificial and fattening and instead consume food that is full of fats such as butter, cheese, nuts and fish.

In this book, you will learn everything about the keto diet – what it is all about, how it works, what are the benefits, how to follow it and how to keep yourself motivated.

Chapter One: Ketogenic Diet Basics

Ketogenic diet is a diet that places and trains your body to be in a state wherein it primarily uses fat for energy. It achieves this through a natural metabolic process of your body called Ketosis that uses fat to create fuel for your body. A ketogenic diet has many similarities to the Atkins diet and many other low-carb diets. It has been known by several different names like low carb high fat, low carb diet and of course, the ketogenic diet.

The ketogenic diet can be implemented by discarding most of the sugars and starches in your diet and by eating healthy fats, moderate amounts of protein and very low carbs. With little carbohydrates in your diet, your body does not receive enough glucose to keep up with your body's caloric requirements. This eventually results in decreasing blood sugar levels in your body as it uses up glucose for its functions. When you eat foods that are high in carbs, your body automatically produces insulin and glucose. Insulin is made to process the glucose that is in your bloodstream by moving it around the body. Glucose is easy for your body to convert and be used for energy. Therefore, it gets chosen over all other energy sources.

As blood sugar level decreases, it looks for the stored glycogen present in your body and breaks it down to glucose and dissolves it in your blood to be distributed throughout your body. However, glycogen stores would also eventually run out. And when it does, your body would start to use fats as a source of energy for functions in its different parts and produce ketones when the liver processes it. Since glucose is used as the primary energy source, the fat in your body isn't needed and gets stored. With a normal, high carb diet, your body uses glucose as its main form of energy. By lowering the carb intake, the body is put into ketosis. These fats could come from the food that you eat, from your meals or from the fat that your body stores. This is what is called ketosis.

When you hit ketosis, your body starts being very efficient at burning fat to create energy. It turns fat in the liver into ketones that supply energy to the brain. Many studies have shown that a keto diet can help you to improve your health and lose some weight. It can also help with Alzheimer's disease, epilepsy, cancer and diabetes.

The primary advantage of following a ketogenic diet is that it restores the capability of your body to use both fat and glucose as fuel to meet its energy or caloric needs. Your body is designed to use both glucose and fat as fuel. However, due to eating a high carbohydrate diet for most of their lives, many people lack the ability to use fat for the body's energy needs. This results in bodies that have a hard time maintaining a healthy weight and a healthy body fat percentage, both of which contribute to poor health. In fact, even if you are not overweight or obese, you may still have excess visceral fat, which is wrapped around your organs like your liver, pancreas and kidneys.

With a ketogenic diet, your body restores its flexibility to use both glucose and fat as fuel for its energy needs. This flexibility keeps your fat cells, both visceral and subcutaneous (the fat located under your skin and on top of your muscles), in check by using the stored energy found in those fat cells. This would, in turn, reduce the risks of having diseases involved with having high-fat stores, specifically visceral fat:

- Type 2 Diabetes
- Coronary Artery/ Heart Disease
- Colorectal Cancer
- Breast Cancer
- High Cholesterol
- High Blood Pressure
- Metabolic Syndrome
- Alzheimer's Disease
- Stroke

- Dementia

Other than decreasing risks of said diseases, this flexibility contributes to losing excess fat and weight in a manageable manner. Normally, while and after losing some weight, your body would feel less sated after eating the same meal you ate before the weight loss process started.

And in addition to this, you might feel an increase in appetite to compensate especially if you've been depriving yourself. However, when your body is in a state of ketosis, ketones help your body manage the hormones that decrease your satiety after meals and increase your appetite and hunger. With this, you lose weight without fighting your body to gain it back through its natural responses as to what it believes to be starvation.

Moreover, being able to utilize glucose and fat for energy prevents you from experiencing the big swings that affect your mental focus, making you hungry and irritable. When glucose runs out, ketones are readily available to fuel your brain. Even better, ketones give your brain a boost, enabling you to have better focus and concentration.

Lastly, the ketogenic diet has long been used for therapy of epilepsy. This diet has been recommended for children with uncontrolled epilepsy since the 1920's. It only disappeared from popular practice when the anti-seizure medication was made available. However, unlike the anti-seizure medicine currently available, the ketogenic diet does not cause extreme side effects on patients; like drowsiness, reduced concentration, personality changes and reduced brain function.

Starting Information & Tips

The Standard Ketogenic Diet (SKD) means that 70 percent of your diet should be in the form of healthy fats, 25 percent in the form of protein and 5 percent of carbohydrates. The percentages would be based on your daily caloric requirement that is unique for every person. Since you may need to increase your caloric intake due to higher needs, you may increase the percentage of healthy fats in your diet and your body can still achieve ketosis.

Other variations of the ketogenic diet that are tweaked based on certain needs are listed down below:

Targeted Ketogenic Diet (TKD)

This type of ketogenic diet is recommended for those who engage in physical fitness. In TKD, 30 to 60 minutes before exercise, you would eat the entirety of your carbohydrates for the day in one meal. The idea of this approach is to use the energy provided in this carbohydrate meal for your fitness activities before it disrupts your body's state of ketosis.

Cyclic Ketogenic Diet (CKD)

This approach is intended for people who have a high rate of physical activities like athletes and bodybuilders. When following CKD, you switch between a ketogenic diet, and after that you follow it with a few days of high carbohydrate consumption (9 to 12 times the carbohydrates in SKD), more commonly called, "carb loading." This approach takes advantage of the body's response to high blood sugar levels from a high carbohydrate diet, which is to store it in the body's muscles and fat cells. Having this abundance of stored energy and the body able to utilize both glucose and fat for energy, it can use this energy to keep the body going during high rates of physical activity.

High-Protein Ketogenic Diet

This is a method used to ease into a Standard Ketogenic Diet when the weight is beyond the normal levels. In this approach, your protein consumption in an SKD is increased by 10 percent and your fat consumption is reduced by 10 percent. This helps those with obesity to help suppress their appetite and reduce their food intake.

Restricted Ketogenic Diet:

This method was successfully used for a brain tumor patient. In this approach, carbohydrate and calorie intake are restricted for your body to deplete glycogen stores and to start producing ketones. Since cancer cells can only feed on glucose, they are starved to death while your body thrives on ketones. It starts with a water fasting regimen and proceeds to only have a Ketogenic Diet of 600 calories a day. After two months, ketosis is in full effect and no discernable brain tumor tissue can be detected.

Only the high protein ketogenic and the standard diets have had extensive studies done on them. The targeted and cyclical diets are more advanced and are only used by athletes and bodybuilders. Even though there are several different types of this diet, the standard ketogenic diet has been researched the most and is, therefore, the one that is usually recommended.

The reason why ketogenic diets are effective lies in the functional property of fat adaption. Your body needs to be told that it has to derive its energy from fats. The biggest challenge in this regard is to keep the body programmed to this state, on a regular basis. In order to maintain ketosis, here are a few tips that you must pay heed to.

Tip 1: Drink Enough Water

You must drink a healthy amount of water to maintain a healthy body. This is a fact that all of us know and are told about time and again. However, it has also proven to be the most difficult advice to follow. The modern lifestyle is so consuming that we mostly forget simple things like keeping our bodies hydrated and eating our meals on time. It is a good idea to drink around 4 glasses of water, first thing in the morning and another 4 glasses of water before the clock strikes noon.

Tip 2: Fast Once In A While

Like we said, our bodies fail to use up the fat stores because we never, ever fast. The body is pre-programmed to run ketosis as and when the body starves. Therefore, if you are finding it hard to get your body into ketosis or maintain the ketosis state of the body, you can fast intermittently. Fasting also helps in reducing food intake and manages appetites and cravings, both of which are crucial for your diet plan. However, be sure to go on a low-carb diet for a few days before fasting intermittently. The sudden lack of sugar in the body may land you up in a hypoglycemic state.

A daylong fast can be easily broken down into two phases. The first phase extends from the first meal you consume to the last meal you eat for the day. This is the build-up phase. The second phase, which extends from your last meal for the day to the first meal of the next day, is the cleansing phase. Ideally, the cleansing phase must be longer than the build-up phase.

Whenever you fast, be sure to keep your body hydrated and eat good fats like butter and coconut oil. These additions play an instrumental role in boosting up the ketone production of the body and help to maintain a healthy insulin level.

Tip 3: Add Good Salts

The high insulin levels of the body, when it is in glycolysis, affect the functioning of the kidney in such a manner that the body retains sodium. As a result, the sodium-potassium ratio destabilizes. This is why most people are advised to reduce their sodium intake. On the other hand, when on a ketogenic diet, the insulin levels are normal and the kidney functioning allows sodium excretion more effectively.

As a result, the body needs sodium to ensure proper functioning. Never make the mistake of avoiding salts when running your body on a ketogenic diet. There are several ways by which you can increase the sodium levels of the body. Some of the best ways include having broth, eating sprouted pumpkin seeds, eating cucumber as part of the salad for natural sodium and adding a pinch of salt to almost everything you eat.

Tip 4: Exercise

Regular exercise can play a crucial role in maintaining the ketosis state of the body and avoiding deposition of glucose in body parts. Exercise allows activation of glucose transport molecules that facilitate deposition of glucose in the muscles and liver. Exercises like the ones used for resistance training also facilitate the maintenance of normal blood sugar levels.

It is important to understand in this context that overdoing exercise can result in the release of stress hormones. This, in turn, increases sugar levels of the body and destabilizes the ketosis state of the body. Regular and 'just-enough' exercise can be a great way to keep you on track.

Tip 5: Avoid Too Much Protein

Most regular diet programs recommend higher protein intake. However, excessive protein intake can initiate what is called gluconeogenesis, which again generates glucose. If you feel that your body is no longer able to maintain the ketosis state, you must take a keen look at the number of proteins that you are consuming. You may have more success with a much lower protein intake.

Tip 6: Choose What You Eat Wisely

Although the ketogenic diet recommends a reduced carbohydrate intake, it is not a good idea to remove carbs from the diet completely. Therefore, the inclusion of starchy vegetables and citric fruit is a good idea. On an odd day when you are off-ketosis, you can consume berries and potatoes. However, when on ketosis, be sure to avoid sweet potato and berry-type fruit completely.

Tip 7: Reduce Stress

Stress is the root cause of most of the problems that your body's face. In fact, an increase in the stress hormones in the body can pull you off ketosis because it increases the sugar levels substantially. Therefore, maintaining a ketosis state can be an uphill task if you are going through stressful times in your life. Managing stress is an important facet of the ketogenic diet. Adopt strategies that keep your stress levels in check if you wish to make your ketogenic diet work. In line with this objective, having adequate amounts of daily sleep and maintaining a stable lifestyle is also essential.

Who should follow this diet?

The keto diet is known in popular discourse only for weight loss, but it's about much more. In this section, we will look at who should follow this diet -

Epileptic Patients

The ketogenic diet was originally developed in the early 1900s as a means of controlling seizures in children. Fasting was long a treatment in treating epilepsy and doctors found that a high-fat diet helped mimic the metabolic response of fasting. They began treating epileptic children by feeding them a diet in which up to 90% of the calories came from fat and found a marked reduction in the seizures. Half of the children fed a ketogenic diet had a reduced number of seizures and about one in seven had a complete elimination of seizures altogether.

Some studies suggest that the ketones created by the ketogenic diet are the reason it is successful in treating epilepsy. Others believe that the depletion of glucose is the reason for its success. Whatever the reason, it has proven to be effective when medication has not.

The ketogenic diet, especially when used to treat seizures, is very intense and highly controlled and can be difficult for children to follow. Doctors usually only recommend it after multiple rounds of medication have proven unsuccessful. However, many of the epileptic children who are put on the ketogenic diet for two years or longer experience a reduction or elimination of seizures, even after they cease eating it. It does not seem to have the same effect in treating epileptic teenagers and adults, possibly because it is so strict and difficult to follow. However, they can still be treated with it as long as they are willing to follow it exactly.

The ketogenic diet for epilepsy is stricter than the ketogenic diet that many people are adhering to boost their health. Rather than a 70% fat this one requires 90% fats. Side effects can include stunted growth, constipation, kidney stones, weight loss and weaker bones. If the side effects become too much, a less intense but possibly less-effective diet, such as modified Atkins, can be implemented instead.

When an epileptic patient is starting out on the ketogenic diet, he or she may need to spend a few days in the hospital for monitoring to see what effects the diet is having. Close medical monitoring will be required, including keeping a food diary, corresponding with a dietitian and getting tested every one to three months. Hyper-vigilance for carbs is required, as they can show up in some very unexpected places. For example, most kinds of toothpaste and mouthwashes contain carbs.

Parents who place their epileptic children on a ketogenic diet will have to make substantial lifestyle changes. They will have to be able to implement the diet in such a way that the epileptic child does not see it as "unfair". He or she may see siblings enjoying sweets and feel left out. All caregivers, including babysitters, teachers and other family members, will have to be aware of the strict diet. Relatives who may want to "spoil" the child by giving him or her treats at family reunions will have to understand how serious the diet is, as one simple misstep or "cheat" can trigger seizures. Some creative ideas for handling these difficult situations include using treats other than food, such as toys, fun outings, or television time. Before Halloween one year, one dad of an epileptic child on the ketogenic diet sent out a letter to all of the homes in his neighborhood that explained why his son couldn't have candy and included a toy to give him instead. The heartwarming letter went viral.

When a medical professional advises getting off the ketogenic diet in favor of a more traditional diet that includes more carbs and protein, the transition will need to be made gradually. Especially in children, the body has become so adjusted to the ketogenic diet that the metabolic changes can be difficult to adapt to.

Type 1 Diabetics

Unlike Type 2 diabetes, Type 1 diabetes is actually an autoimmune disease in which the immune system attacks the pancreas and destroys the beta cells that detect blood sugar and create insulin. As a result, the body's cells are unable to absorb any glucose and blood sugar can build up to dangerously high levels. Type 1 diabetics usually must administer insulin through injections and constantly monitor their blood sugar levels to make sure they are within a safe range. While many people are diagnosed with it as children, half of those diagnosed are over the age of 30.

There are many complications that people with Type 1 diabetes can experience, possibly as a result of the autoimmune dysfunction rather than insulin deficiency. High blood pressure and blood sugar levels can lead to eye damage, such as diabetic retinopathy, nerve damage, kidney damage and heart disease.

The challenge in successfully responding to Type 1 diabetes is not only regulating blood sugar and insulin levels but also dealing with the autoimmune problems that can lead to further complications.

Lifestyle is the most important factor in managing Type 1 diabetes. Avoiding sugar, getting regular exercise, being consistent with insulin injections and being aware of the symptoms of impending problems are some of the most crucial things. Lowering blood sugar, thereby lowering the need for insulin, can be very effective at managing the disease.

The ketogenic diet can be a powerful way of lowering blood sugar in patients with Type 1 diabetes. Many find that they are able to reduce their need for insulin by up to 80% or more.

When following a ketogenic diet with Type 1 diabetes, the person must be absolutely all in. There are no cheats allowed, as just one cheat meal can put the body in a dangerous, potentially deadly state known as ketoacidosis. This occurs when ketones build up in the blood, causing it to become more acidic.

The ketones, which are naturally present on the ketogenic diet, can build up to dangerously high levels as they react with the blood sugar. Diabetics on the ketogenic diet should closely monitor their ketone and glucose levels and remain carefully under a doctor's supervision.

Type 1 diabetics may need to follow a modified version of the ketogenic diet, which is more strictly controlled but more suited to the disease.

Type 2 Diabetics

Type 2 diabetes, also known as adult diabetes, is oftentimes the result of lifestyle choices that lead to chronically high levels of blood sugar, thereby leading to insulin resistance. While Type 1 diabetes is caused by the inability of the body to create insulin, Type 2 diabetes is the result of it being unable to use insulin. Increasingly unhealthy lifestyle choices are leading to children being diagnosed with Type 2 diabetes, whereby it was previously unheard of in people under the age of 50.

Diet, exercise and close monitoring of insulin levels are key to managing Type 2 diabetes. Complete lifestyle overhauls have led some people to completely reverse the symptoms and no longer need medication. The most obvious benefit is that the lowered blood sugar leads to less dependence on insulin.

The conundrum created by applying the ketogenic diet to Type 2 diabetes is that because so many people with the disease are overweight or obese, adopting a high-fat diet seems to be counterintuitive. After all, fat is a much more concentrated source of calories than carbs or protein, so it should actually lead to weight gain and exacerbate the person's health problems. However, that is a myth based on a misunderstanding of calories and the complex chemistry involved in metabolism. The fact is that not all calories are created equal and healthy fats, as opposed to carbs, can actually decrease your appetite so that you end up consuming fewer calories. Additionally, the decreased production of ghrelin, the hunger hormone and the increased production of leptin and amylin, the satiety hormones, generated by the state of ketosis further restrict the calorie intake.

As with Type 1 diabetes, people with Type 2 diabetes are at risk of developing ketoacidosis, so constant monitoring of blood sugar and ketones is important. Additionally, the ketogenic diet should be followed under a doctor's supervision.

Early-Stage Alzheimer's Patients

One of the biggest health concerns today is the risk of developing Alzheimer's disease. Alzheimer's seems to have a bit of a genetic component and is also linked with lifestyle factors. As previously mentioned, some researchers have come to call it Type 3 Diabetes because of its connection with insulin resistance and a buildup of glucose in the brain.

Preliminary studies, both in animal and human trials, indicate that the ketogenic diet is effective at restoring normal brain metabolism in people with early-stage Alzheimer's disease. It reduces and can even eliminate the buildup of unabsorbed glucose that leads to cell death while providing the brain with the superior energy provided by ketones. Ketones are able to provide all of the nutrients necessary for optimal brain function. At optimal levels they do not build up in the bloodstream, leading to the creation of the dangerous plaques and tangles that cause neurodegeneration.

As yet, there is no indication that the ketogenic diet can reverse Alzheimer's disease once it has begun. However, results so far are promising. Research over the past few decades has revealed that the brain has a high level of plasticity, meaning that neurons are able to regenerate, grow and adapt to changing needs. Ketones may be able to tap into this plasticity to help halt Alzheimer's in its tracks and future research into treatment for Alzheimer's will focus heavily on ketones.

People who are diagnosed with Alzheimer's disease tend to be older, usually over the age of 60, so implementing the changes required by the ketogenic diet can be difficult. Additionally, maintaining the person's lifestyle as much as possible is seen as a cornerstone in caring for someone with Alzheimer's, as consistency and normalcy can help deal with the emotional challenges that people with the disease face. Getting Alzheimer's patients to establish a ketogenic diet can be very difficult and will require the complete commitment of all caregivers.

People, who are at risk of developing Alzheimer's disease, because of preexisting insulin resistance, genetic factors, or environmental factors, may benefit from the ketogenic diet. It may prevent the brain decay that is characteristic of the disease.

Parkinson's Patients

Parkinson's disease is a neurodegenerative disorder caused by abnormal levels of the hormone dopamine. The dopamine-creating neurons die and the loss of dopamine results in the characteristic tremors that people with Parkinson's experience. Additionally, they deal with problems such as depression, lack of clarity, forgetfulness and loss of physical function. The disease is progressive, so it gets worse over time. Medications are available to help manage the symptoms, but there is no cure.

Dysfunction in the mitochondria is believed to be a cause of the death of the dopamine-creating neurons, which leads to Parkinson's. The previous chapter already discussed the role of ketones in protecting and enhancing the mitochondria, so from this perspective, ketones may play a role in helping to treat Parkinson's patients. Preliminary studies in animals have shown that the ketogenic diet can improve mitochondrial function. In humans, a preliminary study has shown that one month on the ketogenic diet leads to decreased tremors, elevated mood, improved gait and increased energy.

People who are diagnosed with Parkinson's disease tend to be older, so implementing the intense lifestyle changes required by the ketogenic diet can be quite difficult. Those who participated in the preliminary testing had trouble staying on it and several quit, despite the potential for treatment. A gradual transition to the ketogenic diet may be helpful in maintaining it.

If you want to listen to the full audio book then buy it on www.amazon.com. Search for - Intermittent fasting: Beginners Guide To Weight Loss For Men And Women With Intermittent Fasting by Rogan Jones

Thank you.

Made in the USA
Columbia, SC
24 January 2020